NEW YORK REVIEW BOOKS
CLASSICS

# THE ONE-STRAW REVOLUTION

MASANOBU FUKUOKA (1913–2008) was born and raised on the Japanese island of Shikoku. He was the oldest son of a rice farmer who was also the local mayor. Fukuoka studied plant pathology and worked for three years as a produce inspector in the customs office in Yokohama. But in 1938 he returned to his village home determined to put his ideas about natural farming into practice. During World War II, he worked for the Japanese government as a researcher on food production, managing to avoid military service until the final few months of the war. After the war, he returned to his birthplace to devote himself wholeheartedly to farming. And in 1975, distressed by the effects of Japan's post-war modernization, Fukuoka wrote *The One-Straw Revolution*. In his later years, Fukuoka was involved with several projects to reduce desertification throughout the world. He remained an active farmer until well into his eighties, and continued to give lectures until only a few years before his death at the age of ninety-five. Fukuoka is also the author of *The Natural Way of Farming* and *The Road Back to Nature*. In 1988 he received the Magsaysay Award for Public Service.

FRANCES MOORE LAPPÉ is author or co-author of sixteen books, including *Diet for a Small Planet* and *Getting a Grip: Clarity, Creativity, and Courage in a World Gone Mad*. She has co-founded three organizations, including the Institute for Food and Development Policy and, more recently, the Small Planet Institute, which she leads with her daughter Anna Lappé. In 1987, she received the Right Livelihood Award, also called the "Alternative Nobel." She has received seventeen honorary doctorates and has been a visiting scholar at MIT.

# THE ONE-STRAW REVOLUTION

*An Introduction to Natural Farming*

MASANOBU FUKUOKA

*Edited by*

LARRY KORN

*Preface by*

WENDELL BERRY

*Introduction by*

FRANCES MOORE LAPPÉ

NEW YORK REVIEW BOOKS

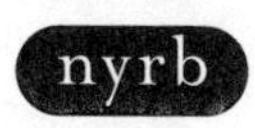


*New York*

THIS IS A NEW YORK REVIEW BOOK
PUBLISHED BY THE NEW YORK REVIEW OF BOOKS
435 Hudson Street, New York, NY 10014
www.nyrb.com



Translated from the Japanese by Larry Korn, Chris Pearce, and Tsune Kurosawa

Published in Japan as *Shizen Noho Wara Ippon No Kakumei* by Shunju-sha Publishers, Tokyo

The publisher wishes to thank Michiyo Shibuya and Larry Korn for their assistance in the preparation of this volume.

Library of Congress Cataloging-in-Publication Data
Fukuoka, Masanobu.
[Shizen noho wara ippon no kakumei. English]
The one-straw revolution : an introduction to natural farming / by Masanobu Fukuoka ; translated from the Japanese by Larry Korn, Chris Pearce, and Tsune Kurosawa ; preface by Wendell Berry ; introduction by Frances Moore Lappé ; with a new afterword by the author.
p. cm. — (New York Review Books classics)
Originally published: Emmaus, Pa. : Rodale Press, 1978.
Includes bibliographical references.
ISBN 978-1-59017-313-8 (alk. paper)
1. No-tillage. 2. Organic farming. 3. No-tillage—Japan. 4. Organic farming—Japan. I. Title. II. Title: Introduction to natural farming. III. Series.
S604.F8413 2009
631.5'84—dc22
2008053698

ISBN 978-1-59017-313-8

Printed in the United States of America
on 30% post-consumer recycled paper.
20 19 18 17 16 15 14 13

# Contents

## III



## IV



## V

# Introduction

It was 1970, and the extent to which our species—supposedly the most intelligent—had failed as steward of the planet had only begun to sink in on me. At age twenty-six, in my first big "ah-ha" moment, I was struck by the realization that we humans had actively created the food scarcity we claimed to fear. We were (and still are) feeding more than a third of the world's grain to livestock, which return to us only a fraction of those nutrients. I was seized with curiosity—why would any species disrupt the source of its own nourishment, its very survival? The next year I published *Diet for a Small Planet.* Could food, I wondered in that book and in subsequent writings, be humanity's pathway to sanity?

Not many years later, Masanobu Fukuoka's volume, now in your hands, swept across the West; it spoke directly to many who had come of age in the sixties and who were now eager to move beyond protest to practical solutions. I was one. True, we'd not yet heard of global climate change and certainly the end of oil seemed imponderably far off; but the dangers of chemical farming were becoming evident to many. We wanted to believe there was another way to nourish ourselves.

*The One-Straw Revolution* we received as an empowering testament to one person's courage to reject the common wisdom that laboratory, narrowly profit-driven science was the salvation of farming. Instead, Fukuoka taught that the best methods of food cultivation are those aligned with nature, which on a practical level means minimal soil disruption (no tilling or weeding) and no application of chemicals (be they fertilizers or pesticides). Back then, the book fortified a budding movement of back-to-the-landers, but today its message is vastly more pertinent: for while the movement to align farming with nature is burgeoning and has spawned various systems—all generally referred to as "organic"—still dominant and spreading globally is the destructive track. It gains strength from the corporate-propagated argument that without massive petrochemicals and soil disruption, we will certainly starve. As a result, pesticide use per acre has quadrupled since my youth and large-scale, fossil-fuel, corporate-monopoly-dependent farming continues to displace traditional practices worldwide.

Today the dangers of petrochemical agriculture are widely known and about two-thirds of Americans say they've tried "organic" food. Even so, the myth remains that organically raised produce is inevitably more expensive than food produced with the benefit of chemicals and must therefore be a luxury, impractical for the masses. Even many who are deeply engaged in sustainability movements revert to the idea of "lack" or of doing without in order to save the environment. Fukuoka, by contrast, encourages us to trust nature's bounty; in *The One-Straw Revolution* he describes how his yields rivaled those of neighboring farms that used the dominant technologies of the day. And in recent years his experience has been widely validated: it is estimated that low- or no-till practices are currently being used to farm 250 million acres of land worldwide, and in 2007 a University of Michigan study projected that overall food availability could increase by about half if the whole world moved to ecologically sane farming.

The assumption that confronting scarcity is an immutable fact of human existence, I believe, has led to the paradox we see today: life-stunting overwork and deprivation for the majority alongside life-stunting overwork and surfeit for the minority. So Fukuoka's message is more deeply radical than simply encouraging farmers to forego tilling or spraying; it cuts to the core of our understanding of ourselves and our place on this earth. He assures us that as we come to experience nature's patterns we can let go of our fear of scarcity.

While Fukuoka does have his list of "do nots," *The One-Straw Revolution* is ultimately about having more not less. Nature can do the work we have unnecessarily taken on ourselves, so what Fukuoka terms "natural farming" is *less* labor intensive. Successful farming is about realizing more leisure in which to experience the richest of relationships, about living in ways that are "gentle and easy." We can enjoy "sitting back" and even being "lazy," writes Fukuoka. To make his point he tells of visiting ancient temples in which Japanese farmers of a bygone era left Haiku they'd composed during their three months of winter leisure. Today, he notes, farmers' three months of leisure have shrunk to days. There is no time to write poetry.

Fukuoka tells us that truly successful agriculture requires not so much arduous labor as awareness, observation, connection, and persistence. Today's agribusiness companies lure farmers to their products by promising that by applying them to their fields according to fixed, prescribed schedules, without much thought about their unique circumstances, farmers can be sure of reliable profits. This might be termed "know-nothing" farming—very different from Fukuoka's "do-nothing" farming, which calls on farmers to question conventional practices that may be needless or even harmful: he advocates a curiosity, openness, and willingness to fail, so that we can learn to trust. His is not simple farming but more complex, aligned farming.

Fukuoka also implies that our fixation on control over nature has led us to assume visual order—the straight, weeded rows of uniform fields—is superior farming. If something appears random, we assume it's wrong. It doesn't match our learned aesthetic. But as we come to experience nature as complex patterns of relationships of which we ourselves are part—patterns having nothing to do with the human, visually ordered world—he suggests that we can come to see beneath appearances. Might we, like Fukuoka, find beauty in what we before perceived as distressingly random and untidy?

In a 1982 interview with *Mother Earth News*, Fukuoka said that "the real path to natural farming requires that a person know what *un*adulterated nature is, so that he or she can instinctively understand what needs to be done—and what must not be done—to work in harmony with its processes."

So my wish is that the reissue and rediscovery of this little, hopeful, almost playful book will help us in the twenty-first century shed our fear of lack, fear that has fueled the drive for control over nature through formulaic answers. My wish is that Fukuoka's insights live on, perhaps more potent now, as part of an ecology of liberation, not only of the earth but of our fear-clutched psyches as well.

Frances Moore Lappé

# Preface

Readers who expect this to be a book only about farming will be surprised to find that it is also a book about diet, about health, about cultural values, about the limits of human knowledge. Others, led to it by hearsay of its philosophy, will be surprised to find it full of practical knowhow about growing rice and winter grain, citrus fruit, and garden vegetables on a Japanese farm.

It is exactly because of such habitual expectations—because we have learned to expect people to be specialists and books to have only one subject—that we are in need of *The One-Straw Revolution.* This book is valuable to us because it is *at once* practical and philosophical. It is an inspiring, necessary book about agriculture because it is not *just* about agriculture.

Knowledgeable readers will be aware that Mr. Fukuoka's techniques will not be directly applicable to most American farms. But it would be a mistake to assume that the practical passages of this book are worthless to us for that reason. They deserve our attention because they provide an excellent *example* of what can be done when land, climate, and crops are studied with fresh interest, clear eyes, and the right kind of concern. They are valuable to us also because they are suggestive and inspiring. Any farmer who reads them will find his thoughts lured repeatedly from the page to his own fields, and from there, making connections, to the entire system of American agriculture.

Like many in this country, and sooner than most, Mr. Fukuoka has understood that we cannot isolate one aspect of life from another. When we change the way we grow our food, we change our food, we change society, we change our values. And so this book is about paying attention to relationships, to causes and effects, and it is about being responsible for what one knows.

Those who are familiar with the literature of organic farming will see the similarities between Mr. Fukuoka's career and that of Sir Albert Howard, the founder of the science of organic agriculture in the West. Like Howard, Mr. Fukuoka started as a laboratory scientist, and, like him, soon saw the limitations of the laboratory. Howard moved his work from the laboratory to the farm, and so changed his life, when he realized that responsibility required him to take his own advice before offering it to other people. Mr. Fukuoka determined his own course in the same way: "Eventually I decided to give my thoughts a form, to put them into practice, and so to determine whether my understanding was right or wrong. To spend my life farming . . . this was the course upon which I settled." And he says: "Instead of offering a hundred explanations, would not practicing this philosophy be the best way?" When the specialist decides to take his own advice, and begins to *do* as he *says*, he breaks down the walls of his specialization. We listen to him then as we could not before, because he speaks with authority—not out of knowledge only, but out of knowledge and experience together.

When Mr. Fukuoka speaks of what he calls his "do-nothing" methods of farming, a Westerner might appropriately be reminded of St. Matthew 6:26: "Behold the fowls of the air: for they sow not, neither do they reap, nor gather into barns; yet your heavenly Father feedeth them." The purpose in both instances, I take it, is to warn us of our proper place in the order of things: we did not make either the world or ourselves; we live by using life, not by creating it. But of course a farmer cannot farm without work any more than a bird can find food without searching for it, a fact that Mr. Fukuoka acknowledges with characteristic good humor: "I advocate 'do-nothing' farming, and so many people come, thinking they will find a utopia where one can live without ever having to get out of bed. These people are in for a big surprise." The argument here is not against work; it is against *unnecessary* work. People sometimes work more than they need to for the things that they desire, and some things that they desire they do not need.

And "do-nothing" also refers to the stance that common sense is apt to take in response to expert authority: "'How about *not* doing this? How about *not* doing that?'—that was my way of thinking." This is the instructive contrariness of children and certain old people, who rightly distrust the "sophistication" that goes ahead without asking "What for?"

Mr. Fukuoka is a scientist who is suspicious of science—or of what too often passes for science. This does not mean that he is either impractical or contemptuous of knowledge. His suspicion, indeed, comes from his practicality and from what he knows. Like Sir Albert Howard, Mr. Fukuoka condemns the piecemealing of knowledge by specialization. Like Howard, he wishes to pursue his subject in its wholeness, and he never forgets that its wholeness includes both what he knows and what he does not know. What he fears in modern applied science is its disdain for mystery, its willingness to reduce life to what is known about it and to act on the assumption that what it does not know can safely be ignored. "Nature as grasped by scientific knowledge," he says, "is a nature which has been destroyed; it is a ghost possessing a skeleton, but no soul." Such a passage will recall the similar mistrust voiced in our own tradition in these lines by Wordsworth:

> Our meddling intellect
> Misshapes the beauteous forms of things—
> We murder to dissect.

Mr. Fukuoka's is a science that begins and ends in reverence—in awareness that the human grasp necessarily diminishes whatever it holds. It is not knowledge, he seems to say, that gives us the sense of the whole, but joy, which we may have only by *not* grasping. We find this corrroborated in certain passages in the Gospels, and in William Blake:

> He who binds to himself a joy
> Doth the winged life destroy;
> But he who kisses the joy as it flies
> Lives in eternity's sunrise.

It is this grace that is the origin of Mr. Fukuoka's agricultural insights: "When it is understood that one loses joy and happiness in the effort to possess them, the essence of natural farming will be realized."

And this "natural" farming that has its source and end in reverence is everywhere human and humane. Humans work best when they work for human good, not for the "higher production" or "increased efficiency" which have been the nearly exclusive goals of industrial agriculture. "The ultimate goal of farming," Mr. Fukuoka says, "is not the growing of crops, but the cultivation and perfection of human beings." And he speaks of agriculture as a *way:* "To be here, caring for a small field, in full possession of the freedom and plentitude of each day, every day—this must have been the original way of agriculture." An agriculture that is whole nourishes the whole person, body and soul. We do not live by bread alone.

Wendell Berry

# Editor's Introduction

Near a small village on the island of Shikoku in southern Japan, Masanobu Fukuoka has been developing a method of natural farming which could help to reverse the degenerative momentum of modern agriculture. Natural farming requires no machines, no chemicals, and very little weeding. Mr. Fukuoka does not plow the soil or use prepared compost. He does not hold water in his rice fields throughout the growing season as farmers have done for centuries in the Orient and around the world. The soil of his fields has been left unplowed for over twenty-five years, yet their yields compare favorably with those of the most productive Japanese farms. His method of farming requires less labor than any other. It creates no pollution and does not require the use of fossil fuels.

When I first heard stories about Mr. Fukuoka, I was skeptical. How could it be possible to grow high-yielding crops of rice and winter grains each year simply by scattering seed onto the surface of an unplowed field? There had to be more to it than that.

For several years I had been living with a group of friends on a farm in the mountains north of Kyoto. We used the traditional methods of Japanese agriculture to grow rice, rye, barley, soybeans, and various garden vegetables. Visitors to our farm often spoke of the work of Mr. Fukuoka. None of these people had stayed long enough at his farm to learn the details of his technique, but their talk excited my curiosity.

Whenever there was a lull in our work schedule, I travelled to other parts of the country, stopping at farms and communes, working part-time along the way. On one of these excursions I paid a visit to Mr. Fukuoka's farm to learn about this man's work for myself.

I am not quite sure what I expected him to be like, but after having heard so much about this great teacher, I was somewhat surprised to see that he was dressed in the boots and the work clothes of the average Japanese farmer. Yet his white wispy beard and alert, self-assured manner gave him the presence of a most unusual person.

I stayed at Mr. Fukuoka's farm for several months on that first visit, working in the fields and in the citrus orchard. There, and in the mudwalled huts in evening discussions with other student farmworkers, the details of Mr. Fukuoka's method and its underlying philosophy gradually became clear to me.

Mr. Fukuoka's orchard is located on the hillsides overlooking Matsuyama Bay. This is "the mountain" where his students live and work. Most of them arrive as I did, with a knapsack on their backs, not knowing what to expect. They stay for a few days or a few weeks, and disappear down the mountain again. But there is usually a core group of four or five who have been there for a year or so. Over the years many people, both women and men, have come to stay and work.

There are no modern conveniences. Drinking water is carried in buckets from the spring, meals are cooked at a wood-burning fireplace, and light is provided by candles and kerosene lamps. The mountain is rich with wild herbs and vegetables. Fish and shellfish can be gathered in nearby streams, and sea vegetables from the Inland Sea a few miles away.

Jobs vary with the weather and the season. The workday begins at about eight; there is an hour for lunch (two or three hours during the heat of midsummer); the students return to the huts from their work just before dusk. Besides the agricultural jobs, there are the daily chores of carrying water, cutting firewood, cooking, preparing the hot bath, taking care of the goats, feeding the chickens and collecting their eggs, minding the bee hives, repairing and occasionally constructing new huts, and preparing *miso* (soybean paste) and *tofu* (soybean curd).

Mr. Fukuoka provides 10,000 yen (about $35) a month for the living expenses of the whole community. Most of it is used to buy soy sauce, vegetable oil, and other necessities which are impractical to produce on a small scale. For the rest of their needs, the students must rely entirely on the crops they grow, the resources of the area, and on their own ingenuity. Mr. Fukuoka purposely has his students live in this semi-primitive manner, as he himself has lived for many years, because he believes that this way of life develops the sensitivity necessary to farm by his natural method.

In the area of Shikoku where Mr. Fukuoka lives, rice is grown on the coastal plains and citrus on the surrounding hillsides. Mr. Fukuoka's farm consists of one and a quarter acres of rice fields and twelve and a half acres of mandarin orange orchards. This may not seem like much to a Western farmer, but because all the work is done with the traditional Japanese hand tools, it requires a lot of labor to maintain even so small an acreage.

Mr. Fukuoka works with the students in the fields and in the orchard, but no one knows exactly when he will visit the job site. He seems to have a knack for appearing at times when the students least expect him. He is an energetic man, always chattering about one thing or another. Sometimes he calls the students together to discuss the work they are doing, often pointing out ways in which the job could be accomplished more easily and quickly. At other times he talks about the life cycle of a weed or disease fungus in the orchard, and occasionally he pauses to recall and reflect upon his farming experiences. Besides explaining his techniques, Mr. Fukuoka also teaches the fundamental skills of agriculture. He emphasizes the importance of caring properly for tools and never tires of demonstrating their usefulness.

If the newcomer expected "natural farming" to mean that nature would farm while he sat and watched, Mr. Fukuoka soon taught him that there was a great deal he had to know and do. Strictly speaking, the only "natural" farming is hunting and gathering. Raising agricultural crops is a cultural innovation which requires knowledge and persistent effort. The fundamental distinction is that Mr. Fukuoka farms by cooperating with nature rather than trying to "improve" upon nature by conquest.

Many visitors come to spend only an afternoon, and Mr. Fukuoka patiently shows them around his farm. It is not uncommon to see him striding up the mountain path with a group of ten or fifteen visitors puffing behind. There have not always been so many visitors, however. For years, while he was developing his method, Mr. Fukuoka had little contact with anyone outside his village.

As a young man, Mr. Fukuoka left his rural home and travelled to Yokohama to pursue a career as a microbiologist. He became a specialist in plant diseases and worked for some years in a laboratory as an agricultural customs inspector. It was at that time, while still a young man of twenty-five, that Mr. Fukuoka experienced the realization which was to form the basis of his life's work and which was to be the theme of this book, *The One-Straw Revolution.* He left his job and returned to his native village to test the soundness of his ideas by applying them in his own fields.

The basic idea came to him one day as he happened to pass an old field which had been left unused and unplowed for many years. There he saw healthy rice seedlings sprouting through a tangle of grasses and weeds. From that time on, he stopped flooding his field in order to grow rice. He stopped sowing rice seed in the spring and, instead, put the seed out in the autumn, sowing it directly onto the surface of the field when it would naturally have fallen to the ground. Instead of plowing the soil to get rid of weeds, he learned to control them by a more or less permanent ground cover of white clover and a mulch of rice and barley straw. Once he has seen to it that conditions have been tilted in favor of his crops, Mr. Fukuoka interferes as little as possible with the plant and animal communities in his fields.

Since many Westerners, even farmers, are not familiar with the rotation of rice and winter grain, and because Mr. Fukuoka makes many references to rice-growing in *The One-Straw Revolution*, it may be helpful to say a few words about traditional Japanese agriculture.

Originally rice seed was cast directly onto the flooded river plain during the monsoon season. Eventually the bottomlands were terraced to hold irrigation water even after the seasonal flooding had subsided.

By the traditional method, used in Japan until the end of the Second World War, rice seed is sown onto a carefully prepared starter bed. Compost and manure are distributed over the field, which is then flooded and plowed to a pea-soup consistency. When the seedlings are about eight inches tall, they are transplanted by hand to the field. Working steadily, an experienced farmer can transplant about one-third of an acre in a day, but the job is almost always done by many people working together.

Once the rice has been transplanted, the field is lightly cultivated between the rows. It is then hand-weeded, and often mulched. For three months the field stays flooded, the water standing an inch or more above the surface of the ground. Harvesting is done with a hand sickle. The rice is bundled and hung on wooden or bamboo racks for a few weeks to dry before threshing. From transplanting to harvest, every inch of the field is gone over at least four times by hand.

As soon as the rice harvest is completed, the field is plowed and the soil is shaped into flattened ridges about a foot wide divided by drainage furrows. The seeds of rye or barley are scattered on top of the hills and covered with soil. This rotation was made possible by a well-timed planting schedule and care to keep the fields well supplied with organic matter and essential nutrients. It is remarkable that, using the traditional method, Japanese farmers grew a crop of rice *and* a winter grain crop each year in the same field for centuries without reducing the fertility of the soil.

Though he recognizes many virtues of the traditional farming, Mr. Fukuoka feels that it involves work that is unnecessary. He speaks of his own methods as "do-nothing" farming and says that they make it possible even for a "Sunday farmer" to grow enough food for the whole family. He does not mean, however, that his sort of farming can be done entirely without effort. His farm is maintained by a regular schedule of field chores. What *is* done must be done properly and with sensitivity. Once the farmer has determined that a plot of land should grow rice or vegetables and has cast the seed, he must assume responsibility for maintaining that plot. To disrupt nature and then to abandon her is harmful and irresponsible.

In the fall Mr. Fukuoka sows the seeds of rice, white clover, and winter grain onto the same fields and covers them with a thick layer of rice straw. The barley or rye and the clover sprout up right away; the rice seeds lie dormant until spring.

While the winter grain is growing and ripening in the lower fields, the orchard hillsides become the center of activity. The citrus harvest lasts from mid-November to April.

The rye and barley are harvested in May and spread to dry on the field for a week or ten days. They are then threshed, winnowed, and put into sacks for storage. All of the straw is scattered unshredded across the field as mulch. Water is then held in the field for a short time during the monsoon rains in June to weaken the clover and weeds and to give the rice a chance to sprout through the ground cover. Once the field is drained, the clover recovers and spreads beneath the growing rice plants. From then until harvest, a time of heavy labor for the traditional farmer, the only jobs in Mr. Fukuoka's rice fields are those of maintaining the drainage channels and mowing the narrow walkways between the fields.

The rice is harvested in October. The grain is hung to dry and then threshed. Autumn seeding is completed just as the early varieties of mandarin oranges are becoming ripe and ready for harvest.

Mr. Fukuoka harvests between 18 and 22 bushels (1,100 to 1,300 pounds) of rice per quarter acre. This yield is approximately the same as is produced by either the chemical or the traditional method in his area. The yield of his winter grain crop is often higher than that of either the traditional farmer or the chemical farmer who both use the ridge and furrow method of cultivation.

All three methods (natural, traditional, and chemical) yield comparable harvests, but differ markedly in their effect on the soil. The soil in Mr. Fukuoka's fields improves with each season. Over the past twenty-five years, since he stopped plowing, his fields have improved in fertility, structure, and in their ability to retain water. By the traditional method the condition of the soil over the years remains about the same. The farmer takes yields in direct proportion to the amount of compost and manure he puts in. The soil in the fields of the chemical farmer becomes lifeless and depleted of its native fertility in a short time.

One of the greatest advantages of Mr. Fukuoka's method is that rice can be grown without flooding the field throughout the growing season. Few people have ever thought this possible. It *is* possible, and Mr. Fukuoka maintains that rice grows better this way. His rice plants are strong-stemmed and deeply rooted. The old variety of glutinous rice that he grows has between 250 and 300 grains per head.

The use of mulch increases the soil's ability to retain water. In many places natural farming can completely eliminate the need for irrigation. Rice and other high-yielding crops can therefore be grown in areas not previously thought suitable. Steep and otherwise marginal land can be brought into production without danger of erosion. By means of natural farming, soils already damaged by careless agricultural practices or by chemicals can be effectively rehabilitated.

Plant diseases and insects are present in the fields

and in the orchard, but the crops are never devastated. The damage affects only the weakest plants. Mr. Fukuoka insists that the best disease and insect control is to grow crops in a healthy environment.

The fruit trees of Mr. Fukuoka's orchard are not pruned low and wide for easy harvesting, but are allowed to grow into their distinctive natural shapes. Vegetables and herbs are grown on the orchard slopes with a minimum of soil preparation. During the spring, seeds of burdock, cabbage, radish, soybeans, mustard, turnips, carrots and other vegetables are mixed together and tossed out to germinate in an open area among the trees before one of the long spring rains. This sort of planting obviously would not work everywhere. It works well in Japan where there is a humid climate with rain dependably falling throughout the spring months. The texture of the soil of Mr. Fukuoka's orchard is clayey. The surface layer is rich in organic matter, friable, and retains water well. This is the result of the cover of weeds and clover that has grown in the orchard continuously for many years.

The weeds must be cut back when the vegetable seedlings are young, but once the vegetables have established themselves they are left to grow up with the natural ground cover. Some vegetables go unharvested, the seeds fall, and after one or two generations, they revert to the growing habits of their strong and slightly bitter-tasting wild predecessors. Many of these vegetables grow up completely untended. Once, not long after I came to Mr. Fukuoka's farm, I was walking through a remote section of the orchard and unexpectedly kicked something hard in the tall grass. Stooping to look more closely, I found a cucumber, and nearby I found a squash nestled among the clover.

For years Mr. Fukuoka wrote about his method in

books and magazines, and was interviewed on radio and television, but almost no one followed his example. At that time Japanese society was moving with determination in exactly the opposite direction.

After the Second World War, the Americans introduced modern chemical agriculture to Japan. This enabled the Japanese farmer to produce approximately the same yields as the traditional method, but the farmer's time and labor were reduced by more than half. This seemed a dream come true, and within one generation almost everyone had switched to chemical agriculture.

For centuries Japanese farmers had maintained organic matter in the soil by rotating crops, by adding compost and manure, and by growing cover crops. Once these practices were neglected and fast-acting chemical fertilizer was used instead, the humus was depleted in a single generation. The structure of the soil deteriorated; crops became weak and dependent on chemical nutrients. To make up for reduced human and animal labor, the new system mined the fertility reserves of the soil.

During the past forty years Mr. Fukuoka has witnessed with indignation the degeneration both of the land and of Japanese society. The Japanese followed singlemindedly the American model of economic and industrial development. The population shifted as farmers migrated from the countryside into the growing industrial centers. The rural village where Mr. Fukuoka was born and where the Fukuoka family has probably lived for 1,400 years or more now stands at the edge of the advancing suburbs of Matsuyama City. A national highway with its litter of *sake* bottles and trash passes through Mr. Fukuoka's rice fields.

Although he does not identify his philosophy with any particular religious sect or organization, Mr.

Fukuoka's terminology and teaching methods are strongly influenced by Zen Buddhism and Taoism. He will sometimes also quote from the Bible and bring up points of Judeo-Christian philosophy and theology to illustrate what he is saying or to stimulate discussion.

Mr. Fukuoka believes that natural farming proceeds from the spiritual health of the individual. He considers the healing of the land and the purification of the human spirit to be one process, and he proposes a way of life and a way of farming in which this process can take place.

It is unrealistic to believe that, in his lifetime and within current conditions, Mr. Fukuoka could completely realize his vision in practice. Even after more than thirty years his techniques are still evolving. His great contribution is to demonstrate that the daily process of establishing spiritual health can bring about a practical and beneficial transformation of the world.

Today, the general recognition of the long-term dangers of chemical farming has renewed interest in alternative methods of agriculture. Mr. Fukuoka has emerged as a leading spokesman for agricultural revolution in Japan. Since the publication of *The One-Straw Revolution* in October, 1975, interest in natural farming has spread rapidly among the Japanese people.

During the year-and-a-half that I worked at Mr. Fukuoka's, I returned frequently to my farm in Kyoto. Everyone there was anxious to try the new method and gradually more and more of our land was converted to natural farming.

Besides rice and rye in the traditional rotation, we also grew wheat, buckwheat, potatoes, corn, and soybeans by Mr. Fukuoka's method. To plant corn and other row crops which germinate slowly, we poked a hole in the soil with a stick or a piece of bamboo and dropped a seed into each hole. We interplanted the corn with soybeans by the same method or by wrapping the seeds in clay pellets and scattering them onto the field. Then we mowed the ground cover of weeds and white clover, and covered the field with straw. The clover came back, but only after the corn and soybeans were well established.

Mr. Fukuoka was able to help by making some suggestions, but we had to adjust the method by trial and error to our various crops and local conditions. We knew from the start that it would take more than just a few seasons, both for the land and our own spirits, to change over to natural farming. The transition has become an on-going process.

Larry Korn

# Notes on the Translation

A literal translation from one language to another would be challenging enough, but to retain the flavor and cultural context of the original as well, is even more difficult. In particular, Japanese is more subtle than English in expressing the kind of spiritual experiences and philosophical teachings which are found in this book. Some terms, such as "discriminating" and "non-discriminating" knowledge, "no-mind," and "do-nothing" have no English equivalent, and so have been rendered literally with additional explanation provided in notes.

It is a common teaching device among Oriental philosophers to use paradox, illogic, and apparent contradiction to help break habitual patterns of thought. Such passages are not necessarily to be taken either literally or figuratively, but rather as exercises to open the consciousness to perception beyond the reach of the intellect.

The Japanese, *mugi,* translated as "winter grain," includes wheat, rye, and barley. The growing methods for these grains are similar, except that wheat generally takes a few weeks longer to mature. Rye and barley are much more commonly grown in Japan because wheat is not ready for harvest until the middle of the Japanese rainy season.

The Japanese, *mikan,* is translated as citrus. The most common Oriental citrus is the mandarin orange. While many varieties of mandarin oranges are grown in Japan, the most common is a small orange fruit very much like our familiar tangerine.

Where context requires, the precise winter grain and citrus varieties are given.

The translation of *The One-Straw Revolution* was begun at Mr. Fukuoka's farm, and under his supervision in Spring, 1976. It is not a verbatim translation. Sections of other works by Mr. Fukuoka, as well as parts of conversations with him, have been included in the text.

L. K.

無

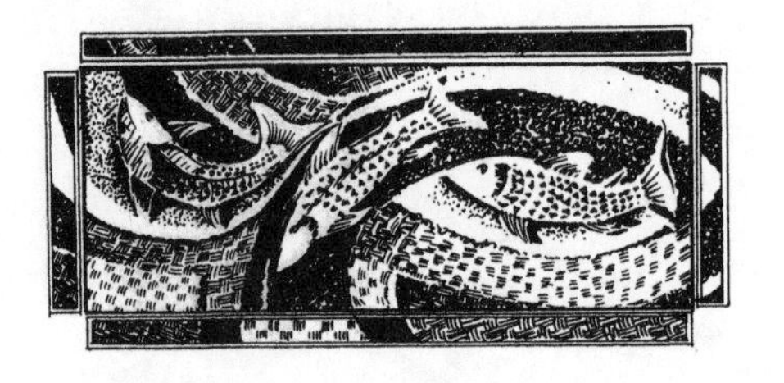

*This translation has been a communal effort by the student workers on the mountain.*

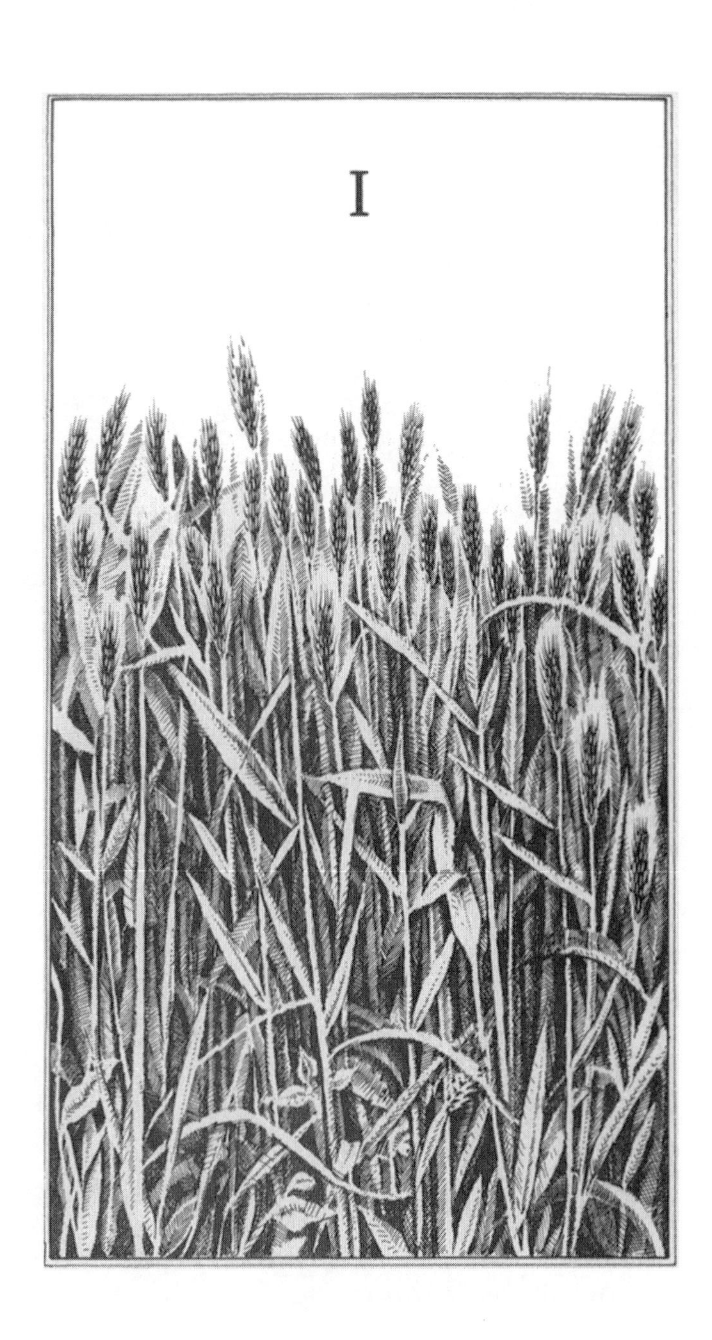
I

## Look at this Grain

I believe that a revolution can begin from this one strand of straw. Seen at a glance, this rice straw may appear light and insignificant. Hardly anyone would believe that it could start a revolution. But I have come to realize the weight and power of this straw. For me, this revolution is very real.

Take a look at these fields of rye and barley. This ripening grain will yield about 22 bushels (1,300 pounds) per quarter acre. I believe this matches the top yields in Ehime Prefecture. And if this equals the best yield in Ehime Prefecture, it could easily equal the top harvest in the whole country since this is one of the prime agricultural areas in Japan. And yet these fields have not been plowed for twenty-five years.

To plant, I simply broadcast rye and barley seed on separate fields in the fall, while the rice is still standing. A few weeks later I harvest the rice and spread the rice straw back over the fields.

It is the same for the rice seeding. This winter grain will be cut around the 20th of May. About two weeks before the crop has fully matured, I broadcast rice seed over the rye and barley. After the winter grain has been harvested and the grains threshed, I spread the rye and barley straw over the field.

I suppose that using the same method to plant rice and winter grain is unique to this kind of farming. But there is an easier way. As we walk over to the next field, let me point out that the rice there was sown last fall at the same time as the winter grain. The whole year's planting was finished in that field by New Year's Day.

You might also notice that white clover and weeds are growing in these fields. Clover seed was sown among the rice plants in early October, shortly before the rye and barley. I do not worry about sowing the weeds—they reseed themselves quite easily.

So the order of planting in this field is like this: in early October clover is broadcast among the rice; winter grain then follows in the middle of the month.

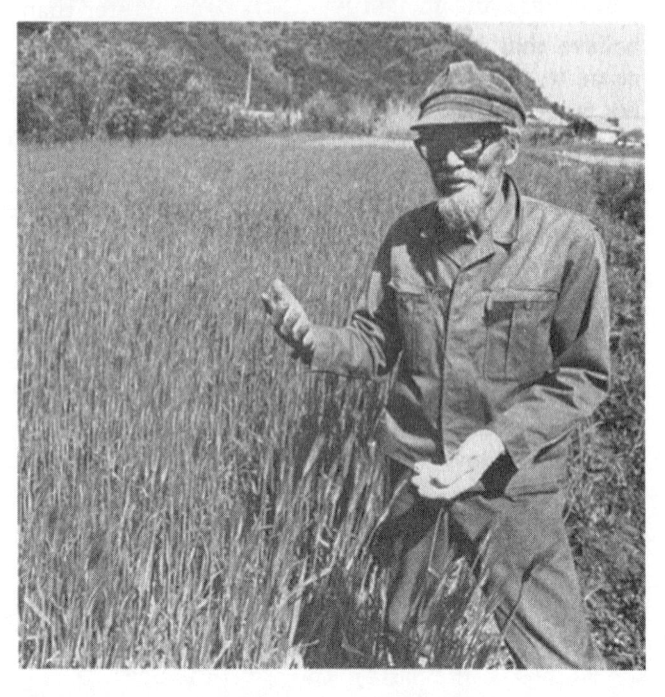

"And yet these fields have not been plowed for twenty-five years."

In early November, the rice is harvested, and then the next year's rice seed is sown and straw laid across the field. The rye and barley you see in front of you were grown this way.

In caring for a quarter-acre field, one or two people can do all the work of growing rice and winter grain in a matter of a few days. It seems unlikely that there could be a simpler way of raising grain.

This method completely contradicts modern agricultural techniques. It throws scientific knowledge and traditional farming know-how right out the window. With this kind of farming, which uses no machines, no prepared fertilizer and no chemicals, it is possible to attain a harvest equal to or greater than that of the average Japanese farm. The proof is ripening right before your eyes.

# Nothing at All

Recently people have been asking me why I started farming this way so many years ago. Until now I have never discussed this with anyone. You could say there was no way to talk about it. It was simply—how would you say it—a shock, a flash, one small experience that was the starting point.

That realization completely changed my life. It is nothing you can really talk about, but it might be put something like this: "Humanity knows nothing at all. There is no intrinsic value in anything, and every action is a futile, meaningless effort." This may seem preposterous, but if you put it into words, that is the only way to describe it.

This "thought" developed suddenly in my head when I was still quite young. I did not know if this insight, that all human understanding and effort are of no account, was valid or not, but if I examined these thoughts and tried to banish them, I could come up with nothing within myself to contradict them. Only the certain belief that this was so burned within me.

It is generally thought that there is nothing more splendid than human intelligence, that human beings are creatures of special value, and that their creations and accomplishments as mirrored in culture and history are wondrous to behold. That is the common belief, anyway.

Since what I was thinking was a denial of this, I was unable to communicate my view to anyone. Eventually I decided to give my thoughts a form, to put them into practice, and so to determine whether my understanding was right or wrong. To spend my life farming, growing rice and winter grain—this was the course upon which I settled.

And what was this experience that changed my life?

Forty years ago, when I was twenty-five years old, I was working for the Yokohama Customs Bureau in the Plant Inspection Division. My main job was to inspect incoming and outgoing plants for disease-carrying insects. I was fortunate to have a good deal of free time, which I spent in the research laboratory, carrying out investigations in my specialty of plant pathology. This laboratory was located next to Yamate Park and looked down on Yokohama harbor from the bluff. Directly in front of the building was the Catholic Church, and to the east was the Ferris Girls' School. It was very quiet, all in all the perfect environment for carrying on research.

The laboratory pathology researcher was Eiichi Kurosawa. I had studied plant pathology under Makoto Okera, a teacher at Gifu Agricultural High School, and received guidance from Suehiko Igata of the Okayama Prefecture Agricultural Testing Center.

I was very fortunate to be a student of Professor Kurosawa. Although he remained largely unknown in the academic world, he is the man who isolated and raised in culture the fungus which causes *bakanae* disease in rice. He became the first to extract the plant growth hormone, gibberellin, from the fungus culture. This hormone, when a small amount is absorbed by the young rice plants, has the peculiar effect of causing the plant to grow abnormally tall. When given in excess, however, it brings about the opposite reaction, causing the plant's growth to be retarded. No one took much notice of this discovery in Japan, but overseas it became a topic of active research. Soon thereafter, an American made use of gibberellin in developing the seedless grape.

I regarded Kurosawa-san* as my own father, and with his guidance, built a dissection microscope and devoted myself to research on decay-causing resin diseases in the trunk, branches and fruit of American and Japanese citrus trees.

Looking through the microscope, I observed fungus cultures, crossbred various fungi and created new disease-causing varieties. I was fascinated with my work. Since the job required deep, sustained concentration, there were times when I actually fell unconscious while working in the lab.

This was also a time of youthful high spirits and I did not spend all of my time shut up in the research room. The place was the port city of Yokohama, no better spot to fool around and have a good time. It was during that time that the following episode occurred. Intent, and with camera in hand, I was strolling by the wharf and caught sight of a beautiful woman. Thinking that she would make a great subject for a photograph, I asked her to pose for me. I helped her onto the deck of the foreign ship anchored there, and asked her to look this way and that and took several pictures. She asked me to send her copies when the photos were ready. When I asked where to send them, she just said, "To Ofuna," and left without mentioning her name.

After I had developed the film, I showed the prints to a friend and asked if he recognized her. He gasped and said, "That's Mieko Takamine, the famous

---

*-*san* is a formal title of address in Japanese used for both men and women.

movie star!" Right away, I sent ten enlarged prints to her in Ofuna City. Before long, the prints, autographed, were returned in the mail. There was one missing, however. Thinking about this later, I realized that it was the close-up profile shot I had taken; it probably showed some wrinkles in her face. I was delighted and felt I had caught a glimpse into the feminine psyche.

At other times, clumsy and awkward though I was, I frequented a dance hall in the Nankingai area. One time I caught sight there of the popular singer, Noriko Awaya, and asked her to dance. I can never forget the feeling of that dance, because I was so overwhelmed by her huge body that I could not even get my arm around her waist.

In any event, I was a very busy, very fortunate young man, spending my days in amazement at the world of nature revealed through the eyepiece of the microscope, struck by how similar this minute world was to the great world of the infinite universe. In the evening, either in or out of love, I played around and enjoyed myself. I believe it was this aimless life, coupled with fatigue from overwork, that finally led to fainting spells in the research room. The consequence of all this was that I contracted acute pneumonia and was placed in the pneumothorax treatment room on the top floor of the Police Hospital.

It was winter and through a broken window the wind blew swirls of snow around the room. It was warm beneath the covers, but my face was like ice. The nurse would check my temperature and be gone in an instant.

As it was a private room, people hardly ever looked in. I felt I had been put out in the bitter cold, and suddenly plunged into a world of solitude and loneliness. I found myself face to face with the fear of death. As I think about it now, it seems a useless fear, but at the time, I took it seriously.

I was finally released from the hospital, but I could not pull myself out of my depression. In what had I placed my confidence until then? I had been unconcerned and content, but what was the nature of that complacency? I was in an agony of doubt about the nature of life and death. I could not sleep, could not apply myself to my work. In nightly wanderings above the bluff and beside the harbor, I could find no relief.

One night as I wandered, I collapsed in exhaustion on a hill overlooking the harbor, finally dozing against the trunk of a large tree. I lay there, neither asleep nor awake, until dawn. I can still remember that it was the morning of the 15th of May. In a daze I watched the harbor grow light, seeing the sunrise and yet somehow not seeing it. As the breeze blew up from below the bluff, the morning mist suddenly disappeared. Just at that moment a night heron appeared, gave a sharp cry, and flew away into the distance. I could hear the flapping of its wings. In an instant all my doubts and the gloomy mist of my confusion vanished. Everything I had held in firm conviction, everything upon which I had ordinarily relied was swept away with the wind. I felt that I understood just one thing. Without my thinking about them, words came from my mouth: "In this world there is nothing at all. . . ." I felt that I understood nothing.*

I could see that all the concepts to which I had been clinging, the very notion of existence itself, were empty fabrications. My spirit became light and clear. I was dancing wildly for joy. I could hear the small birds chirping in the trees, and see the distant waves glistening in the rising sun. The leaves danced green

---

*To "understand nothing," in this sense, is to recognize the insufficiency of intellectual knowledge.

and sparkling. I felt that this was truly heaven on earth. Everything that had possessed me, all the agonies, disappeared like dreams and illusions, and something one might call "true nature" stood revealed.

I think it could safely be said that from the experience of that morning my life changed completely.

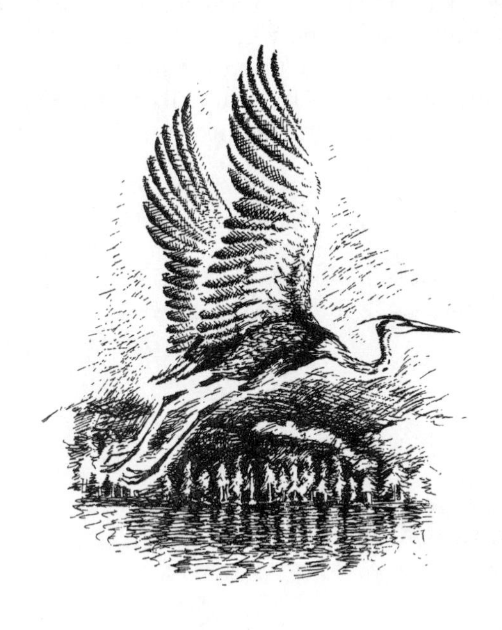

Despite the change, I remained at root an average, foolish man, and there has been no change in this from then to the present time. Seen from the outside, there is no more run-of-the-mill fellow than I, and there has been nothing extraordinary about my daily life. But the assurance that I know this one thing has not changed since that time. I have spent thirty years, forty years, testing whether or not I have been mistaken, reflecting as I went along, but not once have I found evidence to oppose my conviction.

That this realization in itself has great value does not mean that any special value is attached to me. I remain a simple man, just an old crow, so to speak. To the casual observer I may seem either humble or arrogant. I tell the young people up in my orchard again and again not to try to imitate me, and it really angers me if there is someone who does not take this advice to heart. I ask, instead, that they simply live in nature and apply themselves to their daily work. No, there is nothing special about me, but what I have glimpsed is vastly important.

## Returning to the Country

On the day following this experience, May 16th, I reported to work and handed in my resignation on the spot. My superiors and friends were amazed. They had no idea what to make of this. They held a farewell party for me in a restaurant above the wharf, but the atmosphere was a bit peculiar. This young man who had, until the previous day, gotten along well with everyone, who did not seem particularly dissatisfied with his work, who, on the contrary, had wholeheartedly dedicated himself to his research, had suddenly announced that he was quitting. And there I was, laughing happily.

At that time I addressed everyone as follows, "On this side is the wharf. On the other side is Pier 4. If you think there is life on this side, then death is on the other. If you want to get rid of the idea of death, then you should rid yourself of the notion that there is life on this side. Life and death are one."

When I said this everyone became even more concerned about me. "What's he saying? He must be out of his mind," they must have thought. They all saw me off with rueful faces. I was the only one who walked out briskly, in high spirits.

At that time my roommate was extremely worried about me and suggested that I take a quiet rest, perhaps out on the Boso Peninsula. So I left. I would have gone anywhere at all if someone had asked me. I boarded the bus and rode for many miles gazing out at the checkered pattern of fields and small villages along the highway. At one stop, I saw a small sign which read, "Utopia." I got off the bus there and set out in search of it.

On the coast there was a small inn and, climbing the cliff, I found a place with a truly wonderful view. I stayed at the inn and spent the days dozing in the tall grasses overlooking the sea. It may have been a few days, a week, or a month, but anyway I stayed there for some time. As the days passed my exhilaration dimmed, and I began to reflect on just what had happened. You could say I was finally coming to myself again.

I went to Tokyo and stayed for a while, passing the days by walking in the park, stopping people on the street and talking to them, sleeping here and there. My friend was worried and came to see how I was getting along. "Aren't you living in some dream world, some world of illusion?" he asked. "No," I replied, "it's you who are living in the dream world." We both thought, "I am right and you are in the dream world." When my friend turned to say good-bye, I answered with something like, "Don't say good-bye. To part is just to part." My friend seemed to have given up hope.

I left Tokyo, passed through the Kansai area* and came as far south as Kyushu. I was enjoying myself, drifting from place to place with the breeze. I challenged a lot of people with my conviction that everything is meaningless and of no value, that everything returns to nothingness.

But this was too much, or too little, for the everyday world to conceive. There was no communi-

---

* Osaka, Kobe, Kyoto.

cation whatsoever. I could only think of this concept of non-usefulness as being of great benefit to the world, and particularly the present world which is moving so rapidly in the opposite direction. I actually wandered about with the intention of spreading the word throughout the whole country. The outcome was that wherever I went I was ignored as an eccentric. So I returned to my father's farm in the country.

My father was growing tangerines at that time and I moved into a hut on the mountain and began to live a very simple, primitive life. I thought that if here, as a farmer of citrus and grain, I could actually demonstrate my realization, the world would recognize its truth. Instead of offering a hundred explanations, would not practicing this philosophy be the best way? My method of "do-nothing"* farming began with this thought. It was in the 13th year of the present emperor's reign, 1938.

I settled myself on the mountain and everything went well up to the time that my father entrusted me with the richly-bearing trees in the orchard. He had already pruned the trees to "the shape of sake cups" so that the fruit could easily be harvested. When I left them abandoned in this state, the result was that the branches became intertwined, insects attacked the trees and the entire orchard withered away in no time.

My conviction was that crops grow themselves and should not have to be grown. I had acted in the belief that everything should be left to take its natural course, but I found that if you apply this way of thinking all at once, before long things do not go so well. This is abandonment, not "natural farming."

---

*With this expression Mr. Fukuoka draws attention to his method's comparative ease. This way of farming requires hard work, especially at the harvest, but far less than other methods.

My father was shocked. He said I must rediscipline myself, perhaps take a job somewhere and return when I had pulled myself back together. At that time my father was headman of the village, and it was hard for the other members of the community to relate to his eccentric son, who obviously could not get along with the world, living as he did back in the mountains. Moreover, I disliked the prospect of military service, and as the war was becoming more and more violent, I decided to go along humbly with my father's wishes and take a job.

At that time technical specialists were few. The Kochi Prefecture Testing Station heard about me, and it came about that I was offered the post of Head Researcher of Disease and Insect Control. I imposed upon the kindness of Kochi Prefecture for almost eight years. At the testing center I became a supervisor in the scientific agriculture division, and in research devoted myself to increasing wartime food productivity. But actually during those eight years, I was pondering the relationship between scientific and natural agriculture. Chemical agriculture, which utilizes the products of human intelligence, was reputed to be superior. The question which was always in the back of my mind was whether or not natural agriculture could stand up against modern science.

When the war ended I felt a fresh breeze of freedom, and with a sigh of relief I returned to my home village to take up farming anew.

## Toward a Do-Nothing Farming

For thirty years I lived only in my farming and had little contact with people outside my own community. During those years I was heading in a straight line toward a "do-nothing" agricultural method.

The usual way to go about developing a method is to ask "How about trying this?" or "How about trying that?" bringing in a variety of techniques one upon the other. This is modern agriculture and it only results in making the farmer busier.

My way was opposite. I was aiming at a pleasant, natural way of farming* which results in making the work easier instead of harder. "How about *not* doing this? How about *not* doing that?"—that was my way of thinking. I ultimately reached the conclusion that there was no need to plow, no need to apply fertilizer, no need to make compost, no need to use insecticide. When you get right down to it, there are few agricultural practices that are really necessary.

The reason that man's improved techniques seem to be necessary is that the natural balance has been so badly upset beforehand by those same techniques that the land has become dependent on them.

---

*Farming as simply as possible within and in cooperation with the natural environment, rather than the modern approach of applying increasingly complex techniques to remake nature entirely for the benefit of human beings.

This line of reasoning not only applies to agriculture, but to other aspects of human society as well. Doctors and medicine become necessary when people create a sickly environment. Formal schooling has no intrinsic value, but becomes necessary when humanity creates a condition in which one must become "educated" to get along.

Before the end of the war, when I went up to the citrus orchard to practice what I then thought was natural farming, I did no pruning and left the orchard to itself. The branches became tangled, the trees were attacked by insects and almost two acres of mandarin orange trees withered and died. From that time on the question, "What is the natural pattern?" was always in my mind. In the process of arriving at the answer, I wiped out another 400 trees. Finally I felt I could say with certainty: "This is the natural pattern."

To the extent that trees deviate from their nat-

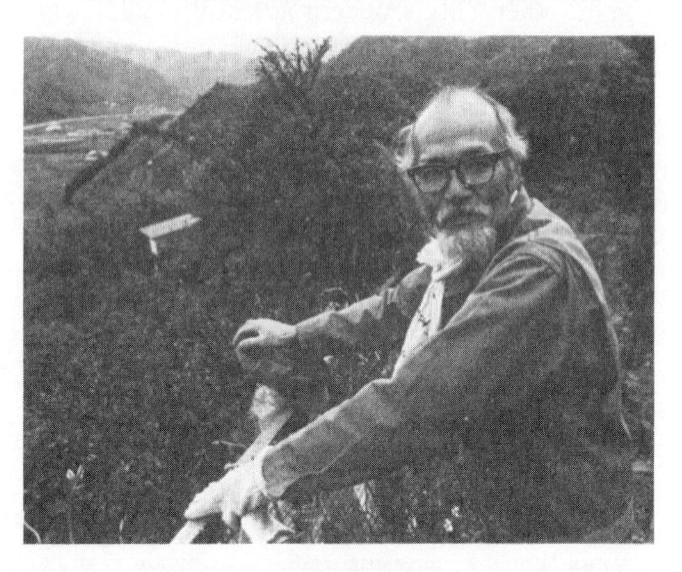

"For thirty years I lived only in my farming. . . ."

ural form, pruning and insect extermination become necessary; to the extent that human society separates itself from a life close to nature, schooling becomes necessary. In nature, formal schooling has no function.

In raising children, many parents make the same mistake I made in the orchard at first. For example, teaching music to children is as unnecessary as pruning orchard trees. A child's ear catches the music. The murmuring of a stream, the sound of frogs croaking by the riverbank, the rustling of leaves in the forest, all these natural sounds are music—true music. But when a variety of disturbing noises enter and confuse the ear, the child's pure, direct appreciation of music degenerates. If left to continue along that path, the child will be unable to hear the call of a bird or the sound of the wind as songs. That is why music education is thought to be beneficial to the child's development.

The child who is raised with an ear pure and clear may not be able to play the popular tunes on the violin or the piano, but I do not think this has anything to do with the ability to hear true music or to sing. It is when the heart is filled with song that the child can be said to be musically gifted.

Almost everyone thinks that "nature" is a good thing, but few can grasp the difference between natural and unnatural.

If a single new bud is snipped off a fruit tree with a pair of scissors, that may bring about disorder which cannot be undone. When growing according to the natural form, branches spread alternately from the trunk and the leaves receive sunlight uniformly. If this sequence is disrupted the branches come into conflict, lie one upon another and become tangled, and the leaves wither in the places where the sun cannot penetrate. Insect damage develops. If the tree is not pruned the following year more withered branches will appear.

Human beings with their tampering do something wrong, leave the damage unrepaired, and when the adverse results accumulate, work with all their might to correct them. When the corrective actions appear to be successful, they come to view these measures as splendid accomplishments. People do this over and over again. It is as if a fool were to stomp on and break the tiles of his roof. Then when it starts to rain and the ceiling begins to rot away, he hastily climbs up to mend the damage, rejoicing in the end that he has accomplished a miraculous solution.

It is the same with the scientist. He pores over books night and day, straining his eyes and becoming nearsighted, and if you wonder what on earth he has been working on all that time—it is to become the inventor of eyeglasses to correct nearsightedness.

## Returning to the Source

Leaning against the long handle of my scythe, I pause in my work in the orchard and gaze out at the mountains and the village below. I wonder how it is that people's philosophies have come to spin faster than the changing seasons.

The path I have followed, this natural way of farming, which strikes most people as strange, was first interpreted as a reaction against the advance and reckless development of science. But all I have been doing, farming out here in the country, is trying to show that humanity knows nothing. Because the world is moving with such furious energy in the opposite direction, it may appear that I have fallen behind the times, but I firmly believe that the path I have been following is the most sensible one.

During the past few years the number of people interested in natural farming has grown considerably. It seems that the limit of scientific development has been reached, misgivings have begun to be felt, and the time for reappraisal has arrived. That which was viewed as primitive and backward is now unexpectedly seen to be far ahead of modern science. This may seem strange at first, but I do not find it strange at all.

I discussed this with Kyoto University Professor Iinuma recently. A thousand years ago agriculture was practiced in Japan without plowing, and it was not until the Tokugawa Era 300-400 years ago that shallow cultivation was introduced. Deep plowing came to Japan with Western agriculture. I said that in coping with the problems of the future the next generation would return to the non-cultivation method.

To grow crops in an unplowed field may seem at first a regression to primitive agriculture, but over the years this method has been shown in university laboratories and agricultural testing centers across the country to be the most simple, efficient, and up-to-date method of all. Although this way of farming disavows modern science, it now has come to stand in the forefront of modern agricultural development.

I presented this "direct seeding non-cultivation winter grain/rice succession" in agricultural journals twenty years ago. From then on it appeared often in print and was introduced to the public at large on radio and television programs many times, but nobody paid much attention to it.

Now suddenly, it is a completely different story. You might say that natural farming has become the rage. Journalists, professors, and technical researchers are flocking to visit my fields and the huts up on the mountain.

Different people see it from different points of view, make their own interpretations, and then leave. One sees it as primitive, another as backward, someone else considers it the pinnacle of agricultural achievement, and a fourth hails it as a breakthrough into the future. In general, people are only concerned with whether this kind of farming is an advance into the future or a revival of times past. Few are able to grasp correctly that natural farming arises from the unmoving and unchanging center of agricultural development.

To the extent that people separate themselves

from nature, they spin out further and further from the center. At the same time, a centripetal effect asserts itself and the desire to return to nature arises. But if people merely become caught up in reacting, moving to the left or to the right, depending on conditions, the result is only more activity. The non-moving point of origin, which lies outside the realm of relativity, is passed over, unnoticed. I believe that even "returning-to-nature" and anti-pollution activities, no matter how commendable, are not moving toward a genuine solution if they are carried out solely in reaction to the overdevelopment of the present age.

Nature does not change, although the way of viewing nature invariably changes from age to age. No matter the age, natural farming exists forever as the wellspring of agriculture.

## One Reason That Natural Farming Has Not Spread

Over the past twenty or thirty years this method of growing rice and winter grain has been tested over a wide range of climates and natural conditions. Almost every prefecture in Japan has run tests comparing yields of "direct seeding non-cultivation" with those of paddy rice growing and the usual ridge and furrow rye and barley cultivation. These tests have produced no evidence to contradict the universal applicability of natural farming.

And so one may ask why this truth has not spread. I think that one of the reasons is that the world has become so specialized that it has become impossible for people to grasp anything in its entirety. For example, an expert in insect damage prevention from the Kochi Prefectural Testing Center came to inquire why there were so few rice leaf-hoppers in my fields even though I had not used insecticide. Upon investigating the habitat, the balance between insects and their natural enemies, the rate of spider propagation and so on, the leaf-hoppers were found to be just as scarce in my fields as in the Center's fields, which are sprayed countless times with a variety of deadly chemicals.

The professor was also surprised to find that while the harmful insects were few, their natural predators were far more numerous in my fields than in the sprayed fields. Then it dawned on him that the fields were being maintained in this state by means of a natural balance established among the various insect communities. He acknowledged that if my method were generally adopted, the problem of crop devastation by leaf-hoppers could be solved. He then got into his car and returned to Kochi.

But if you ask whether or not the testing center's soil fertility or crop specialists have come here, the answer is no, they have not. And if you were to suggest at a conference or gathering that this method, or rather non-method, be tried on a wide scale, it is my guess that the prefecture or research station would reply, "Sorry, it's too early for that. We must first carry out research from every possible angle before giving final approval." It would take years for a conclusion to come down.

This sort of thing goes on all the time. Specialists and technicians from all over Japan have come to this farm. Seeing the fields from the standpoint of his own specialty, every one of these researchers has found them at least satisfactory, if not remarkable. But in the five or six years since the professor from the research station came to visit here, there have been few changes in Kochi Prefecture.

This year the agricultural department of Kinki University has set up a natural farming project team in which students of several different departments will come here to conduct investigations. This approach may be one step nearer, but I have a feeling that the next move may be two steps in the opposite direction.

Self-styled experts often comment, "The basic idea of the method is all right, but wouldn't it be more convenient to harvest by machine?" or, "Wouldn't the yield be greater if you used fertilizer or pesticide in certain cases or at certain times?" There are always those who try to mix natural and scientific farming. But this way of thinking completely misses the point. The farmer who moves toward compromise can no longer criticize science at the fundamental level.

Natural farming is gentle and easy and indicates a return to the source of farming. A single step away from the source can only lead one astray.

## Humanity Does Not Know Nature

Lately I have been thinking that the point must be reached when scientists, politicians, artists, philosophers, men of religion, and all those who work in the fields should gather here, gaze out over these fields, and talk things over together. I think this is the kind of thing that must happen if people are to see beyond their specialties.

Scientists think they can understand nature. That is the stand they take. Because they are convinced that they can understand nature, they are committed to investigating nature and putting it to use. But I think an understanding of nature lies beyond the reach of human intelligence.

I often tell the young people in the huts on the mountain, who come here to help out and to learn about natural farming, that anybody can see the trees up on the mountain. They can see the green of the leaves; they can see the rice plants. They think they know what green is. In contact with nature morning and night, they sometimes come to think that they know nature. But when they think they are beginning to understand nature, they can be sure that they are on the wrong track.

Why is it impossible to know nature? That which is conceived to be nature is only the *idea* of nature arising in each person's mind. The ones who see true nature are infants. They see without thinking, straight and clear. If even the names of plants are known, a mandarin orange tree of the citrus family, a pine of the pine family, nature is not seen in its true form.

An object seen in isolation from the whole is not the real thing.

Specialists in various fields gather together and observe a stalk of rice. The insect disease specialist sees only insect damage, the specialist in plant nutrition considers only the plant's vigor. This is unavoidable as things are now.

As an example, I told the gentleman from the research station when he was investigating the relation between rice leaf-hoppers and spiders in my fields, "Professor, since you are researching spiders, you are interested in only one among the many natural predators of the leaf-hopper. This year spiders appeared in great numbers, but last year it was toads. Before that, it was frogs that predominated. There are countless variations."

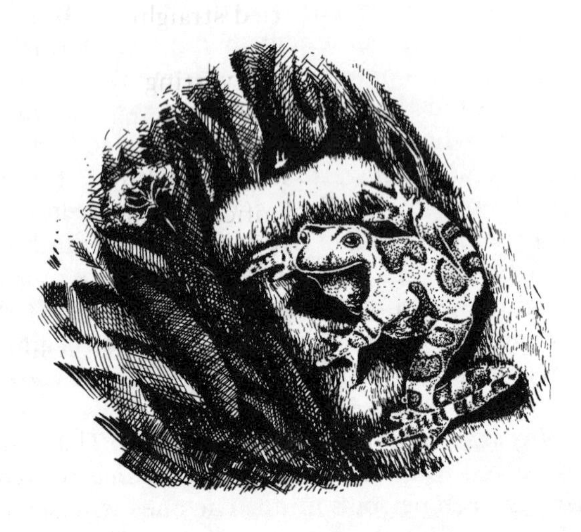

It is impossible for specialized research to grasp the role of a single predator at a certain time within the intricacy of insect inter-relationships. There are seasons when the leaf-hopper population is low because there are many spiders. There are times when a lot of rain falls and frogs cause the spiders to disappear, or when little rain falls and neither leaf-hoppers nor frogs appear at all.

Methods of insect control which ignore the relationships among the insects themselves are truly useless. Research on spiders and leaf-hoppers must also consider the relation between frogs and spiders. When things have reached this point, a frog professor will also be needed. Experts on spiders and leaf-hoppers, another on rice, and another expert on water management will all have to join the gathering.

Furthermore, there are four or five different kinds of spiders in these fields. I remember a few years ago when somebody came rushing over to the house early one morning to ask me if I had covered my fields with a silk net or something. I could not imagine what he was talking about, so I hurried straight out to take a look.

We had just finished harvesting the rice, and overnight the rice stubble and low-lying grasses had become completely covered with spider webs, as though with silk. Waving and sparkling with the morning mist, it was a magnificent sight.

The wonder of it is that when this happens, as it does only once in a great while, it only lasts for a day or two. If you look closely there are several spiders in every square inch. They are so thick on the field that there is hardly any space between them. In a quarter acre there must be how many thousands, how many millions! When you go to look at the field two or three days later, you see that strands of web several yards long have broken off and are waving about in the wind with five or six spiders clinging to each one. It is like when dandelion fluff or pine cone seeds are blown away in the wind. The young spiders cling to the strands and are sent sailing off in the sky.

The spectacle is an amazing natural drama. Seeing this, you understand that poets and artists will also have to join in the gathering.

When chemicals are put into a field, this is all destroyed in an instant. I once thought there would be nothing wrong with putting ashes from the fireplace onto the fields.* The result was astounding. Two or three days later the field was completely bare of spiders. The ashes had caused the strands of web to disintegrate. How many thousands of spiders fell victim to a single handful of this apprently harmless ash? Applying an insecticide is not simply a matter of eliminating the leaf-hoppers together with their natural predators. Many other essential dramas of nature are affected.

The phenomenon of these great swarms of spiders, which appear in the rice fields in the autumn and like escape artists vanish overnight, is still not understood. No one knows where they come from, how they survive the winter, or where they go when they disappear.

And so the use of chemicals is not a problem for the entomologist alone. Philosophers, men of religion, artists and poets must also help to decide whether or not it is permissible to use chemicals in farming, and what the results of using even organic fertilizers might be.

We will harvest about 22 bushels (1,300 pounds) of rice, and 22 bushels of winter grain from each quarter acre of this land. If the harvest reaches 29 bushels,

---

* Mr. Fukuoka makes compost of his wood ashes and other organic household wastes. He applies this to his small kitchen garden.

as it sometimes does, you might not be able to find a greater harvest if you searched the whole country. Since advanced technology had nothing to do with growing this grain, it stands as a contradiction to the assumptions of modern science. Anyone who will come and see these fields and accept their testimony, will feel deep misgivings over the question of whether or not humans know nature, and of whether or not nature can be known within the confines of human understanding.

The irony is that science has served only to show how small human knowledge is.

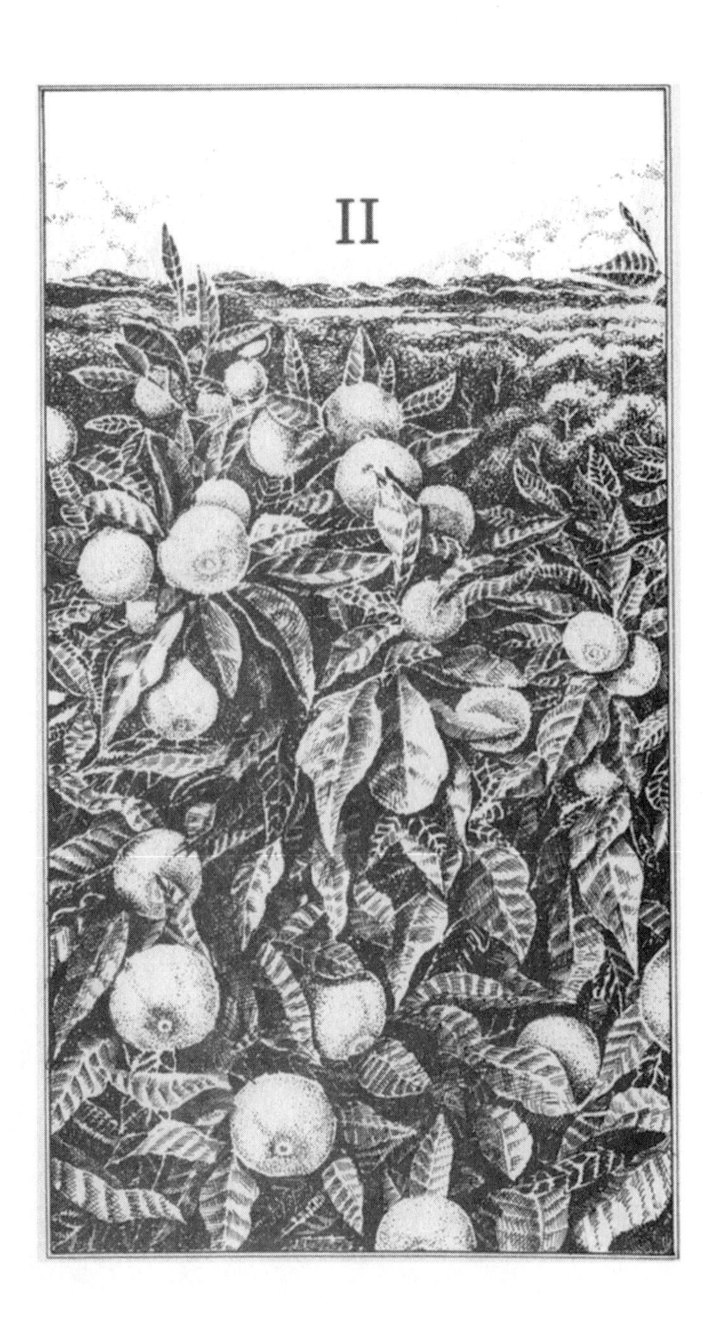
II

# Four Principles of Natural Farming

Make your way carefully through these fields. Dragonflies and moths fly up in a flurry. Honeybees buzz from blossom to blossom. Part the leaves and you will see insects, spiders, frogs, lizards and many other small animals bustling about in the cool shade. Moles and earthworms burrow beneath the surface.

This is a balanced rice field ecosystem. Insect and plant communities maintain a stable relationship here. It is not uncommon for a plant disease to sweep through this area, leaving the crops in these fields unaffected.

And now look over at the neighbor's field for a moment. The weeds have all been wiped out by herbicides and cultivation. The soil animals and insects have been exterminated by poison. The soil has been burned clean of organic matter and microorganisms by chemical fertilizers. In the summer you see farmers at work in the fields, wearing gas masks and long rubber gloves. These rice fields, which have been farmed continuously for over 1,500 years, have now been laid waste by the exploitive farming practices of a single generation.

## Four Principles

The first is NO CULTIVATION, that is, no plowing or turning of the soil. For centuries, farmers have assumed that the plow is essential for growing crops. However, non-cultivation is fundamental to natural farming. The earth cultivates itself naturally by means of the penetration of plant roots and the activity of microorganisms, small animals, and earthworms.

The second is NO CHEMICAL FERTILIZER OR PREPARED COMPOST.* People interfere with nature, and, try as they may, they cannot heal the resulting wounds. Their careless farming practices drain the soil of essential nutrients and the result is yearly depletion of the land. If left to itself, the soil maintains its fertility naturally, in accordance with the orderly cycle of plant and animal life.

The third is NO WEEDING BY TILLAGE OR HERBICIDES. Weeds play their part in building soil fertility and in balancing the biological community. As a fundamental principle, weeds should be controlled, not eliminated. Straw mulch, a ground cover of white clover interplanted with the crops, and temporary flooding provide effective weed control in my fields.

The fourth is NO DEPENDENCE ON CHEMICALS.** From the time that weak plants developed as a result of such unnatural practices as plowing and fertilizing, disease and insect imbalance became a great problem in agriculture. Nature, left alone, is in perfect balance. Harmful insects and plant diseases are always present, but do not occur in nature to an extent which requires the use of poisonous chemicals. The sensible approach to disease and insect control is to grow sturdy crops in a healthy environment.

---

*For fertilizer Mr. Fukuoka grows a leguminous ground cover of white clover, returns the threshed straw to the fields, and adds a little poultry manure.

**Mr. Fukuoka grows his grain crops without chemicals of any kind. On some orchard trees he occasionally uses a machine oil emulsion for the control of insect scales. He uses no persistent or broad-spectrum poisons, and has no pesticide "program."

## Cultivation

When the soil is cultivated the natural environment is altered beyond recognition. The repercussions of such acts have caused the farmer nightmares for countless generations. For example, when a natural area is brought under the plow very strong weeds such as crabgrass and docks sometimes come to dominate the vegetation. When these weeds take hold, the farmer is faced with a nearly impossible task of weeding each year. Very often, the land is abandoned.

In coping with problems such as these, the only sensible approach is to discontinue the unnatural practices which have brought about the situation in

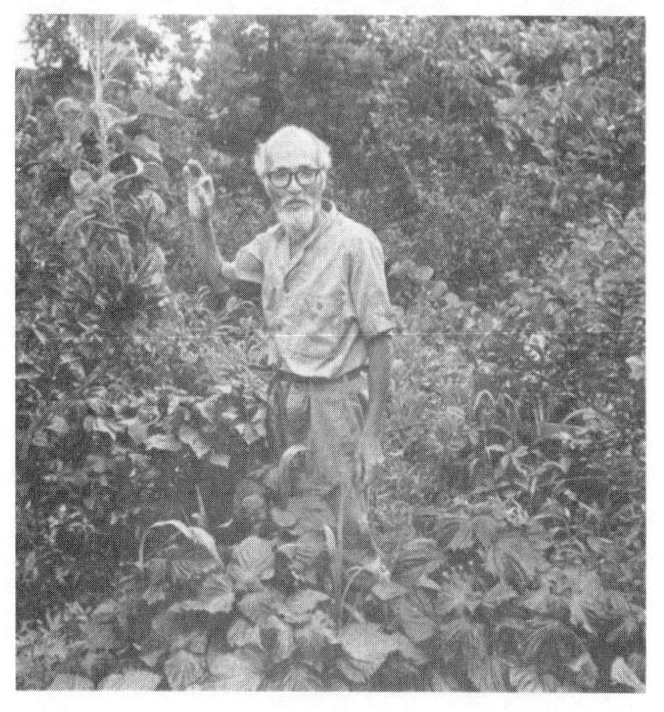

the first place. The farmer also has a responsibility to repair the damage he has caused. Cultivation of the soil should be discontinued. If gentle measures such as spreading straw and sowing clover are practiced, instead of using man-made chemicals and machinery to wage a war of annihilation, then the environment will move back toward its natural balance and even troublesome weeds can be brought under control.

## Fertilizer

I have been known, in chatting with soil fertility experts, to ask, "If a field is left to itself, will the soil's fertility increase or will it become depleted?" They usually pause and say something like, "Well, let's see . . . It'll become depleted. No, not when you remember that when rice is grown for a long time in the same field without fertilizer, the harvest settles at about 9 bushels (525 pounds) per quarter acre. The earth would become neither enriched nor depleted."

These specialists are referring to a cultivated, flooded field. If nature is left to itself, fertility increases. Organic remains of plants and animals accumulate and are decomposed on the surface by bacteria and fungi. With the movement of rainwater, the nutrients are taken deep into the soil to become food for microorganisms, earthworms, and other small animals. Plant roots reach to the lower soil strata and draw the nutrients back up to the surface.

If you want to get an idea of the natural fertility of the earth, take a walk to the wild mountainside sometime and look at the giant trees that grow without fertilizer and without cultivation. The fertility of nature, as it is, is beyond reach of the imagination.

Cut down the natural forest cover, plant Japanese red pine or cedar trees for a few generations, and the soil will become depleted and open to erosion. On the other hand, take a barren mountain with poor, red clay soil, and plant pine or cedar with a ground cover of clover and alfalfa. As the green manure* enriches and softens the soil, weeds and bushes grow up below the trees, and a rich cycle of regeneration is begun. There are instances in which the top four inches of soil have become enriched in less than ten years.

For growing agricultural crops, also, the use of prepared fertilizer can be discontinued. For the most part, a permanent green manure cover and the return of all the straw and chaff to the soil will be sufficient. To provide animal manure to help decompose the straw, I used to let ducks loose in the fields. If they are introduced as ducklings while the seedlings are still young, the ducks will grow up together with the rice. Ten ducks will supply all the manure necessary for a quarter acre and will also help to control the weeds.

I did this for many years until the construction of a national highway made it impossible for the ducks to get across the road and back to the coop. Now I use a little chicken manure to help decompose the straw. In other areas ducks or other small grazing animals are still a practical possibility.

Adding too much fertilizer can lead to problems. One year, right after the rice transplanting, I contracted to rent 1¼ acres of freshly planted rice fields for a period of one year. I ran all the water out of the fields and proceeded without chemical fertilizer, applying only a small amount of chicken manure. Four of the fields developed normally. But in the fifth, no matter what I did, the rice plants came up too thickly and were attacked by blast disease. When I asked the owner about this, he said he had used the field over the winter as a dump for chicken manure.

---

* Ground cover crops such as clover, vetch, and alfalfa which condition and nourish the soil.

Using straw, green manure, and a little poultry manure, one can get high yields without adding compost or commercial fertilizer at all. For several decades now, I have been sitting back, observing nature's method of cultivation and fertilization. And while watching, I have been reaping bumper crops of vegetables, citrus, rice, and winter grain as a gift, so to speak, from the natural fertility of the earth.

## Coping with Weeds

Here are some key points to remember in dealing with weeds:

As soon as cultivation is discontinued, the number of weeds decreases sharply. Also, the varieties of weeds in a given field will change.

If seeds are sown while the preceding crop is still ripening in the field, those seeds will germinate ahead of the weeds. Winter weeds sprout only after the rice has been harvested, but by that time the winter grain already has a head start. Summer weeds sprout right after the harvest of barley and rye, but the rice is already growing strongly. Timing the seeding in such a way that there is no interval between succeeding crops gives the grain a great advantage over the weeds.

Directly after the harvest, if the whole field is covered with straw, the germination of weeds is stopped short. White clover sowed with the grain as a ground cover also helps to keep weeds under control.

The usual way to deal with weeds is to cultivate the soil. But when you cultivate, seeds lying deep in the soil, which would never have germinated otherwise, are stirred up and given a chance to sprout. Furthermore, the quick-sprouting, fast-growing varieties are given the advantage under these conditions. So you might say that the farmer who tries to control weeds by cultivating the soil is, quite literally, sowing the seeds of his own misfortune.

## "Pest" Control

Let us say that there are still some people who think that if chemicals are not used their fruit trees and field crops will wither before their very eyes. The fact of the matter is that by *using* these chemicals, people have unwittingly brought about the conditions in which this unfounded fear may become reality.

Recently Japanese red pines have been suffering severe damage from an outbreak of pine bark weevils. Foresters are now using helicopters in an attempt to stop the damage by aerial spraying. I do not deny that this is effective in the short run, but I know there must be another way.

Weevil blights, according to the latest research, are not a direct infestation, but follow upon the action of mediating nematodes. The nematodes breed within the trunk, block the transport of water and nutrients, and eventually cause the pine to wither and die. The ultimate cause, of course, is not yet clearly understood.

Nematodes feed on a fungus within the tree's trunk. Why did this fungus begin to spread so prolifically within the tree? Did the fungus begin to multiply after the nematode had already appeared? Or did the nematode appear because the fungus was already present? It boils down to a question of which came first, the fungus or the nematode?

Furthermore, there is another microbe about which very little is known, which always accompanies the fungus, and a virus toxic to the fungus. Effect following effect in every direction, the only thing that can be said with certainty is that the pine trees are withering in unusual numbers.

People cannot know what the true cause of the pine blight is, nor can they know the ultimate consequences of their "remedy." If the situation is meddled with unknowingly, that only sows the seeds for the next great catastrophe. No, I cannot rejoice in the knowledge that immediate damage from the weevil has been reduced by chemical spraying. Using agricultural chemicals is the most inept way to deal with problems such as these, and will only lead to greater problems in the future.

These four principles of natural farming (no cultivation, no chemical fertilizer or prepared compost, no weeding by tillage or herbicides, and no dependence on chemicals) comply with the natural order and lead to the replenishment of nature's richness. All my fumblings have run along this line of thought. It is the heart of my method of growing vegetables, grain, and citrus.

## Farming Among the Weeds

Many different kinds of weeds are growing with the grain and clover in these fields. Rice straw spread over the field last fall has already decomposed into rich humus. The harvest will yield about 22 bushels (1,300 pounds) to the quarter acre.

Yesterday, when Professor Kawase, a leading authority on pasture grasses, and Professor Hiroe, who is researching ancient plants, saw the fine spread of barley and green manure in my fields, they called it a wonderful work of art. A local farmer who had expected to see my fields completely overgrown by weeds was surprised to find the barley growing so vigorously among the many other plants. Technical experts have also come here, seen the weeds, seen the watercress and clover growing all around, and have gone away shaking their heads in amazement.

Twenty years ago, when I was encouraging the use of permanent ground cover in fruit orchards, there was not a blade of grass to be seen in fields or orchards anywhere in the country. Seeing orchards such as mine, people came to understand that fruit trees could grow quite well among the weeds and grasses. Today orchards covered with grasses are common throughout Japan and those without grass cover have become rare.

It is the same with fields of grain. Rice, barley,

and rye can be successfully grown while the fields are covered with clover and weeds all year long.

Let me review in greater detail the annual seeding and harvesting schedule in these fields. In early October, before the harvest, white clover and the seeds of fast-growing varieties of winter grain are broadcast among the ripening stalks of rice.* The clover and barley or rye sprout and grow an inch or two by the time the rice is ready to be harvested. During the rice harvest, the sprouted seeds are trampled by the feet of the harvesters, but recover in no time at all. When the threshing is completed, the rice straw is spread over the field.

* White clover is sown about one pound per quarter acre, winter grains 6½ to 13 pounds per quarter acre. For inexperienced farmers or fields with hard or poor soil, it is safer to sow more seed in the beginning. As the soil gradually improves from the decomposing straw and green manure, and as the farmer becomes more familiar with the direct seeding non-cultivation method, the amount of seed can be reduced.

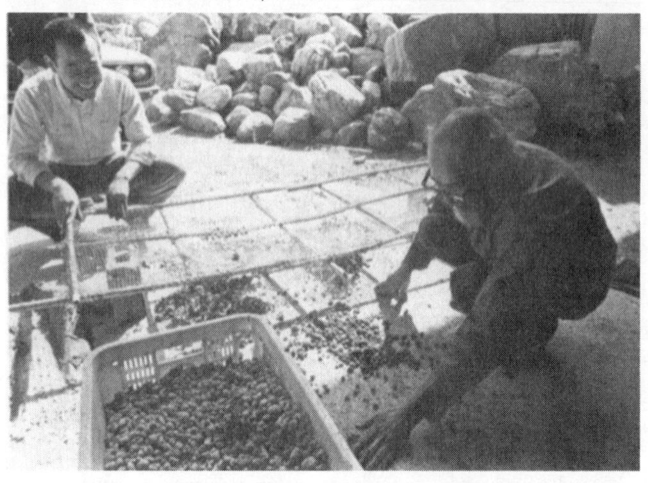

"In one day it is possible to make enough pellets to seed several acres."

If rice is sown in the autumn and left uncovered, the seeds are often eaten by mice and birds, or they sometimes rot on the ground, and so I enclose the rice seeds in little clay pellets before sowing. The seed is spread out on a flat pan or basket and shaken back and forth in a circular motion. Fine powdered clay is dusted over them and a thin mist of water is added from time to time. This forms a tiny pellet about a half inch in diameter.

There is another method for making the pellets.

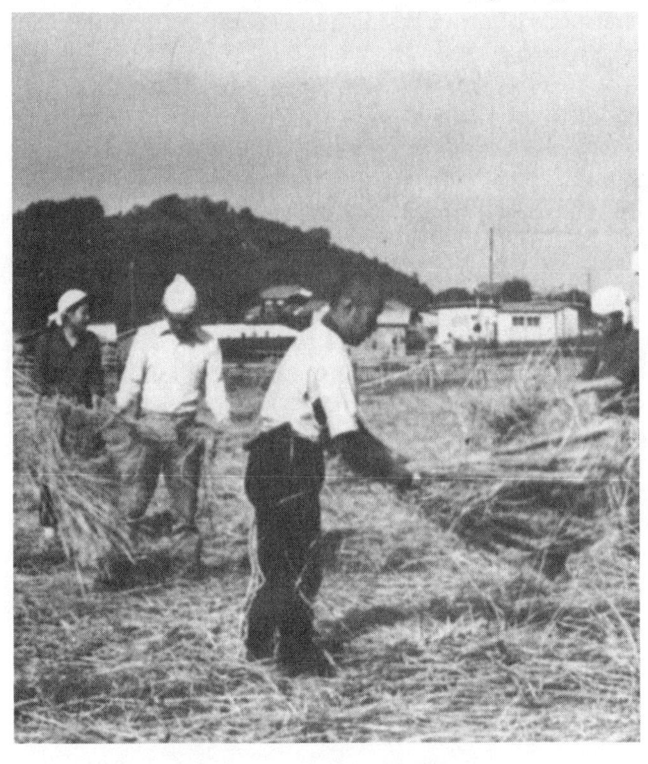

In October, after the rice is harvested and the next year's seed is sown, straw is scattered across the field.

First the unhulled rice seed is soaked for several hours in water. The seeds are removed and mixed with moist clay by kneeding with hands or feet. Then the clay is pushed through a screen of chicken wire to separate it into small clods. The clods should be left to dry for a day or two or until they can be easily rolled between the palms into pellets. Ideally there is one seed in each pellet. In one day it is possible to make enough pellets to seed several acres.

Depending on conditions, I sometimes enclose the seeds of other grains and vegetables in pellets before sowing.

Between mid-November and mid-December is a good time to broadcast the pellets containing the rice seed among the young barley or rye plants, but they can also be broadcast in spring.* A thin layer of chicken manure is spread over the field to help decompose the straw, and the year's planting is complete.

In May the winter grain is harvested. After threshing, all of the straw is scattered over the field.

Water is then allowed to stand in the field for a week or ten days. This causes the weeds and clover to weaken and allows the rice to sprout up through the straw. Rain water alone is sufficient for the plants during June and July; in August fresh water is run through the field about once a week without being allowed to stand. The autumn harvest is now at hand.

Such is the yearly cycle of rice/winter grain cultivation by the natural method. The seeding and harvesting so closely follow the natural pattern that it could be considered a natural process rather than an agricultural technique.

It takes only an hour or two for one farmer to sow

---

*Rice is sown 4½ to 9 pounds per quarter acre. Toward the end of April Mr. Fukuoka checks the germination of the fall-sown seed and broadcasts more pellets as needed. Also see footnote, pg. 42.

the seeds and spread the straw across a quarter acre. With the exception of the job of harvesting, winter grain can be grown single-handedly, and just two or three people can do all the work necessary to grow a field of rice using only the traditional Japanese tools. There is probably no easier, simpler method for growing grain. It involves little more than broadcasting seed and spreading straw, but it has taken me over thirty years to reach this simplicity.

This way of farming has evolved according to the natural conditions of the Japanese islands, but I feel that natural farming could also be applied in other areas and to the raising of other indigenous crops. In areas where water is not so readily available, for example, upland rice or other grains such as buckwheat, sorghum or millet might be grown. Instead of white clover, another variety of clover, alfalfa, vetch

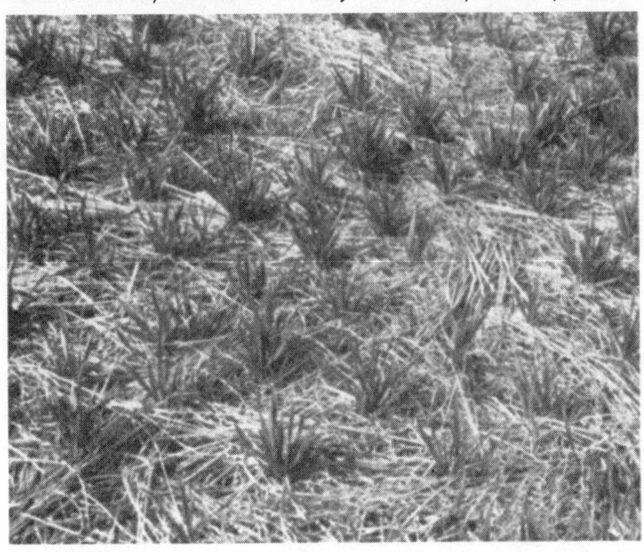

By December the winter grain sprouts through the straw; the rice seeds remain dormant until spring.

or lupine might prove a more suitable field cover. Natural farming takes a distinctive form in accordance with the unique conditions of the area in which it is applied.

In making the transition to this kind of farming, some weeding, composting or pruning may be necessary at first, but these measures should be gradually reduced each year. Ultimately, it is not the growing technique which is the most important factor, but rather the state of mind of the farmer.

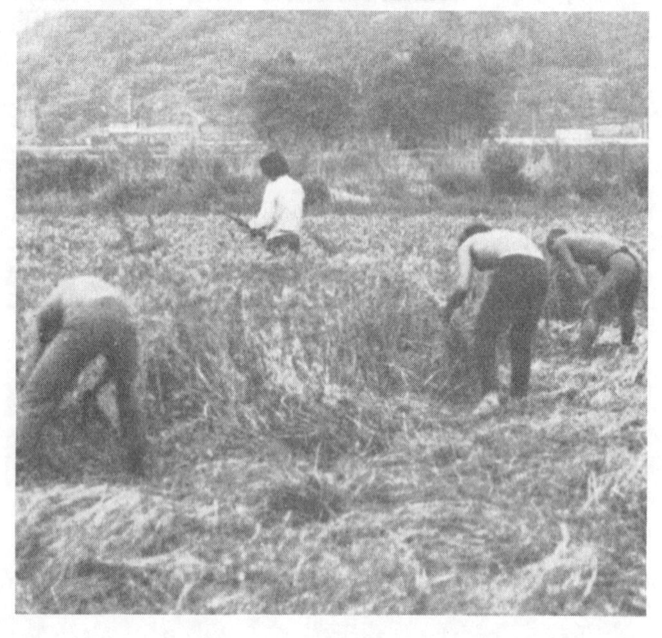

The winter grain is harvested in May. The rice seedlings are trampled by the feet of the harvesters but soon recover.

# Farming with Straw

Spreading straw might be considered rather unimportant, but it is fundamental to my method of growing rice and winter grain. It is connected with everything, with fertility, with germination, with weeds, with keeping away sparrows, with water management. In actual practice and in theory, the use of straw in farming is a crucial issue. This is something that I cannot seem to get people to understand.

## Spreading the Straw Uncut

The Okayama Testing Center is now trying direct seeding rice-growing in 80 percent of its experimental fields. When I suggested that they scatter the straw uncut, they apparently thought this could not be right, and ran the experiments after chopping it up with a mechanical shredder. When I went to visit the testing a few years ago, I found that the fields had been divided into those using shredded straw, uncut straw, and no straw at all. This is exactly what I did for a long time and since the uncut works best, it is uncut straw that I use.

Mr. Fujii, a teacher at Yasuki Agricultural High School in Shimane Prefecture, wanted to try direct seeding and came to visit my farm. I suggested that he spread uncut straw over his field. He returned the next year and reported that the test had failed. After listening carefully to his account, I found that he had laid the straw down straight and neat like a Japanese backyard garden mulch. If you do it like that, the seeds will not germinate well at all. With the straw of rye and barley, too, if it is spread too neatly the rice sprouts will have a hard time getting through. It is best to toss the straw around every which way, just as though the stalks had fallen naturally.

Rice straw works well as a mulch for winter grain, and the straw of winter grain works best for the rice. I want this to be well understood. There are several diseases of rice which will infect the crop if fresh rice straw is applied to the field. These diseases of rice will not infect the winter grain, however, and if the rice straw is spread in the fall, it will be completely decomposed by the time the rice sprouts up the following spring. Fresh rice straw is safe for other grains, as is buckwheat straw, and the straw of other grain species may be used for rice and buckwheat. In general, fresh straw of winter grains, such as wheat, rye, and barley, should not be used as mulch for other winter grains, as disease damage may result.

All of the straw and the hulls which remain after threshing the previous harvest should be returned to the field.

## Straw Enriches the Earth

Scattering straw maintains soil structure and enriches the earth so that prepared fertilizer becomes unnecessary. This, of course, is connected with noncultivation. My fields may be the only ones in Japan which have not been plowed for over twenty years, and the quality of the soil improves with each season. I would estimate that the surface layer, rich in humus, has become enriched to a depth of more than four inches during these years. This is largely the result of returning to the soil everything grown in the field but the grain itself.

## No Need to Prepare Compost

There is no need to prepare compost. I will not say that you do not need compost—only that there is no need to work hard making it. If straw is left lying on the surface of the field in the spring or fall and is covered with a thin layer of chicken manure or duck droppings, in six months it will completely decompose.

To make compost by the usual method, the farmer works like crazy in the hot sun, chopping up the straw, adding water and lime, turning the pile, and hauling it out to the field. He puts himself through all this grief because he thinks it is a "better way." I would rather see people just scattering straw or hulls or woodchips over their fields.

Travelling along the Tokaido line in western Japan I have noticed that the straw is being cut more coarsely than when I first started talking about spreading it uncut. I have to give the farmers credit. But the modern day experts are still saying that it is best to use only so many hundred pounds of straw per quarter acre. Why don't they say to put all the straw back in the field? Looking out the train window, you can see farmers who have cut and scattered about half the straw and cast the rest aside to rot in the rain.

If all the farmers in Japan got together and started to put all the straw back on their fields, the result would be an enormous amount of compost returned to the earth.

## Germination

For hundreds of years farmers have taken great

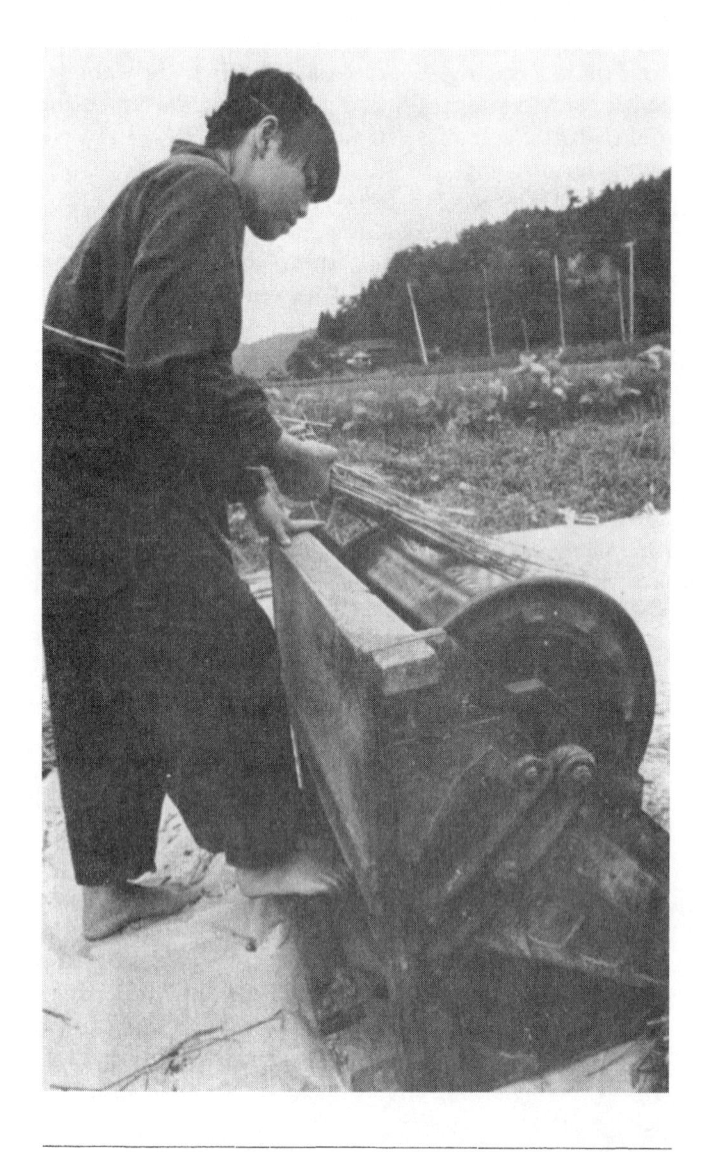

Threshing the crop with the traditional pedal-powered rotating drum (Kyoto). The grains are then winnowed and stored; the straw is returned to the fields.

care in preparing the seed beds for growing strong, healthy rice seedlings. The small beds were tidied up as if they were the family altars. The earth was cultivated, sand and the ashes of burned rice hulls were spread all around, and a prayer was offered that the seedlings would thrive.

It is not unreasonable, then, that the other villagers around here thought I was out of my mind to broadcast seed while the winter grain was still standing in the field, with weeds and bits of decomposing straw scattered everywhere.

Of course the seeds germinate well when sown directly onto a well-turned field, but if it rains and the field turns to mud, you cannot go in and walk around, and the sowing must be postponed. The non-cultivation method is safe on this score, but on the other hand, there is trouble with small animals such as moles, crickets, mice, and slugs who like to eat the seeds. The clay pellet enclosing the seed solves this problem.

In seeding winter grain, the usual method is to sow the seeds and then cover them with soil. If the seeds are set in too deeply, they will rot. I used to drop the seeds into tiny holes in the soil, or into furrows without covering them with soil, but I experienced many failures with both methods.

Lately I have gotten lazy and instead of making furrows or poking holes in the ground, I wrap the seeds in clay pellets and toss them directly onto the field. Germination is best on the surface, where there is exposure to oxygen. I have found that where these pellets are covered with straw, the seeds germinate well and will not rot even in years of heavy rainfall.

## Straw Helps to Cope with Weeds and Sparrows

Ideally, one quarter acre will provide about 900 pounds of barley straw. If all of the straw is spread back over the field, the surface will be completely covered. Even a troublesome weed such as crabgrass, the most difficult problem in the direct seeding non-cultivation method, can be held under control.

Sparrows have caused me a lot of headaches. Direct seeding cannot succeed if there is no reliable way to cope with the birds, and there are many places where direct seeding has been slow to spread for just this reason. Many of you may have the same problem with sparrows, and you will know what I mean.

I can remember times when these birds followed right behind me and devoured all the seeds I had sown even before I had a chance to finish planting the other side of the field. I tried scarecrows and nets and strings of rattling cans, but nothing seemed to work very well. Or if one of these methods happened to work, its effectiveness did not last more than a year or two.

My own experience has shown that by sowing the seed while the preceding crop is still in the field so that they are hidden among grasses and clover, and by spreading a mulch of rice, rye, or barley straw as soon as the mature crop has been harvested, the problem of sparrows can be dealt with most effectively.

I have made a lot of mistakes while experimenting over the years and have experienced failures of all kinds. I probably know more about what can go wrong growing agricultural crops than anyone else in Japan. When I succeeded for the first time in growing rice and winter grain with the non-cultivation method, I felt as joyful as Columbus must have felt when he discovered America.

# Growing Rice in a Dry Field

By the beginning of August, the rice plants in the neighbors' fields are already waist high, while the plants in my fields are only about half that size. People who visit here toward the end of July are always skeptical, and ask, "Fukuoka-san, is this rice going to turn out all right?" "Sure," I answer. "No need to worry."

I do not try to raise tall fast-growing plants with big leaves. Instead, I keep the plants as compact as possible. Keep the head small, do not overnourish the plants, and let them grow true to the natural form of the rice plant.

Usually rice plants three or four feet tall produce luxuriant leaves and give the impression that the plant is going to produce a lot of grain, but it is only the leafy stalks that are growing strongly. Starch production is great but efficiency is low, and so much energy is expended in vegetative growth that not much is left to be stored in the grains. For example, if tall, oversized plants yield 2,000 pounds of straw the yield of rice will be about 1,000-1,200 pounds. For small rice plants, such as those grown in my fields, 2,000 pounds of straw yields 2,000 pounds of rice. In a good harvest the yield of rice from my plants will reach about 2,400 pounds; that is, it will be 20 percent heavier than the straw.

Rice plants grown in a dry field do not grow so tall. Sunlight is received uniformly, reaching to the base of the plants and to the lower leaves. One square inch of leaf is enough to produce six grains of rice. Three or four small leaves are more than enough to produce a hundred grains of rice to the head. I sow a bit thickly and wind up with about 250-300 grain-bearing stalks (20 to 25 plants) per square yard. If you have many sprouts and do not try to grow large plants, you can reap great harvests with no difficulty. This is also true for wheat, rye, buckwheat, oats, millet, and other grains.

Of course the usual method is to keep several inches of water in the paddy throughout the growing season. Farmers have been growing rice in water for so many centuries that most people believe that it cannot be grown any other way. The cultivated varieties of "wet-field" rice are relatively strong if grown in a flooded field, but it is not good for the plant to be grown in this way. Rice plants grow best when the water content in the soil is between 60 and 80 percent of its water-holding capacity. When the field is not flooded plants develop stronger roots and are extremely resistant to attacks by disease and insects.

The main reason for growing rice in a flooded field is to control the weeds by creating an environment in which only a limited variety of weeds can survive. Those which do survive, however, must be pulled by hand or uprooted with a hand weeding tool. By the traditional method, this time-consuming and backbreaking job must be repeated several times in each growing season.

In June, during the monsoon season, I hold water in the field for about one week. Few of the dry-field weeds can survive even so short a period without oxygen, and the clover also withers and turns yellow. The idea is not to kill the clover, but only to weaken it so as to allow the rice seedlings to get established. When the water is drained (as soon as possible) the clover recovers and spreads to cover the field's surface again beneath the growing rice plants. After that, I hardly do anything in the way of water management. For the first half of the season, I do not irrigate at all. Even in years when very little rain falls the soil stays moist below the layer of straw and green manure. In August I let in water a little at a time but never allow it to stand.

If you show a rice plant from my field to a farmer he will know immediately that it looks as a rice plant

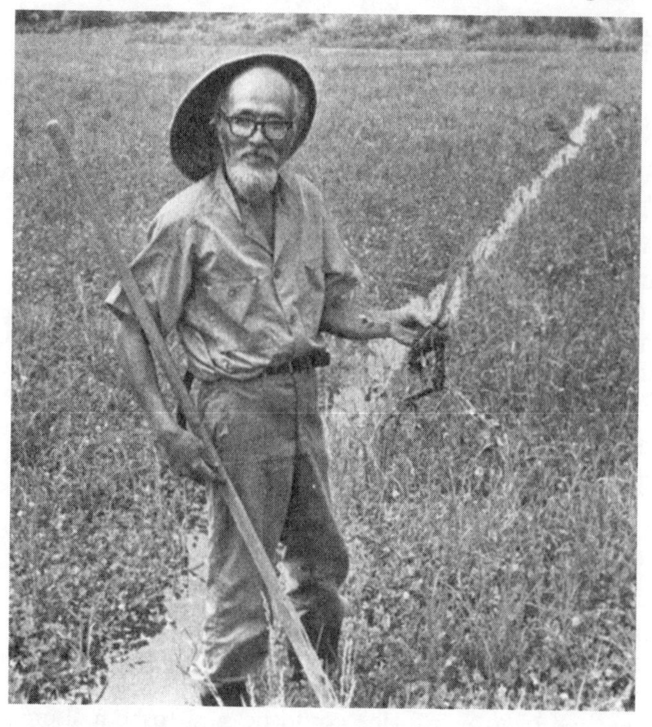

In June water is held in the field to weaken the weeds and clover and allow the rice to sprout through the ground cover.

should and that it has the ideal shape. He will know that the seeds were sprouted naturally and not transplanted, that the plant could not have been grown in a lot of water, and that chemical fertilizer was not applied. Any farmer can tell these things as a matter of course by looking at the overall form of the plant, the shape of the roots, and the spacing of the joints on the main stem. If you understand the ideal form, it is just a matter of how to grow a plant of that shape under the unique conditions of your own field.

I do not agree with Professor Matsushima's idea that it is best when the fourth leaf from the tip of the plant is the longest. Sometimes when the second or third leaf is the longest, you get the best results. If growth is held back while the plant is young, the top leaf or the second leaf often becomes longest and a large harvest is still obtained.

Professor Matsushima's theory is derived from experiments using fragile rice plants grown with fertilizer in a nursery bed and later transplanted. My rice, on the other hand, was grown in accordance with the natural life cycle of the rice plant, just as though it were growing wild. I wait patiently for the plant to develop and mature at its own pace.

In recent years I have been trying out an old variety of glutinous rice from the south. Each seed, sown in fall, produces an average of 12 stalks with about 250 grains per head. With this variety I believe I will one day be able to reap a harvest close to the greatest theoretically obtainable from the solar energy reaching the field. In some areas of my fields harvests of 27½ bushels (1,650 pounds) per quarter acre have already been realized with this variety.

Seen with the doubting eye of the technician, my method of growing rice could be said to be a short-term or provisional result. "If the experiment were continued longer, some sort of problem would certainly show up," he might say. But I have been growing rice in this manner for over twenty years. The yields continue to increase and the soil becomes richer every year.

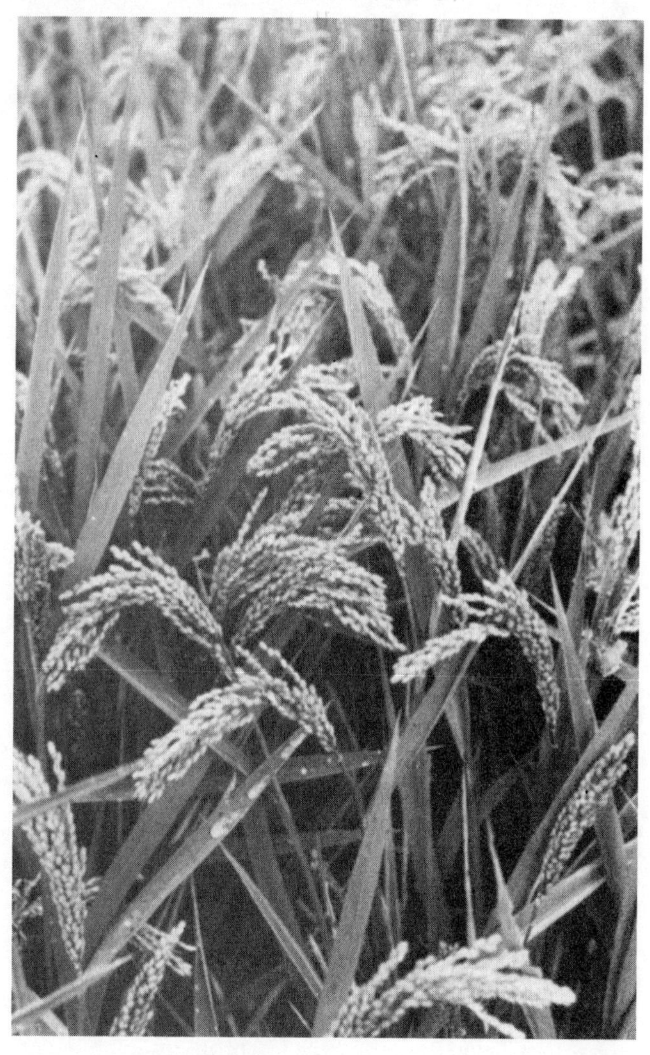

# Orchard Trees

I also grow several varieties of citrus on the hillsides near my home. After the war, when I first began farming, I started with 1¾ acres of citrus orchard and ⅜ acre of rice fields, but now the citrus orchards alone cover 12½ acres. I came by this land by taking over surrounding hillsides which had been abandoned. I then cleared them by hand.

The pine trees on several of those slopes had been clear-cut a few years earlier, and all I did was dig holes in a contour line and plant the citrus seedlings. Sprouts had already appeared from the logged stumps and, as time passed, Japanese pampas grass, cogon grass, and bracken began to thrive. The citrus tree seedlings became lost in a tangle of vegetation.

I cut most of the pine sprouts, but allowed some to grow back for a windbreak. Then I cut back the thicket growth and grassy ground cover and planted clover.

After six or seven years the citrus trees finally bore fruit. I dug away the earth behind the trees to form terraces, and the orchard now appears little different from any other.

Of course I maintained the principles of not cultivating, not using chemical fertilizer, and not using insecticides or weed killers. One interesting thing was that, at first, while the seedlings were growing beneath the resprouted forest trees, there was no evidence of damaging insects such as the common arrowhead scale. Once the thicket and resprouted trees were cut away, the land became less wild and more like an orchard. Only then did these insects appear.

To allow a fruit tree to follow its natural form from the beginning is best. The tree will bear fruit every year and there is no need to prune. A citrus tree follows the same pattern of growth as a cedar or pine, that is, a single central trunk growing straight with branches spreading out alternately. Of course all varieties of citrus do not grow to exactly the same size and shape. The Hassaku and Shaddock varieties grow very tall, winter Unshu mandarin orange trees are short and stocky, the early varieties of Satsuma mandarin orange trees are small at maturity, but each has a single central trunk.

## Do Not Kill the Natural Predators

I think that everyone knows that since the most common orchard "pests," ruby scale and horned wax scale, have natural enemies, there is no need to apply insecticide to keep them under control. At one time the insecticide Fusol was used in Japan. The natural predators were completely exterminated, and the resulting problems still survive in many prefectures. From this experience I think most farmers have come to realize that it is undesirable to eliminate predators because in the long run greater insect damage will result.

As for the mites and scales which do appear, if a solution of machine oil, a chemical relatively harmless to the predators, is diluted 200 to 400 times and is sprayed lightly in midsummer, and the insect communities are left to achieve their natural balance after that, the problem will generally take care of itself. This will not work if an organic phosphorous pesticide has already been used in June or July since the predators are also killed by this chemical.

I am not saying that I advocate the use of so-called harmless "organic" sprays such as salt-garlic solution or machine oil emulsion, nor am I in favor of introducing foreign predator species into the orchard to control troublesome insects. Trees weaken and are attacked by insects to the extent that they deviate from the natural form. If trees are growing along a pattern of unnatural development and are left abandoned in this state, the branches become tangled and insect damage results. I have already told how I wiped out several acres of citrus trees this way.

But if the trees are gradually corrected, they will return at least approximately to their natural form. The trees become stronger and measures to control insects become unnecessary. If a tree is planted carefully and allowed to follow the natural form from the beginning, there is no need for pruning or sprays of any kind. Most seedling trees have been pruned or their roots have been damaged at the nursery before they are transplanted to the orchard, which makes pruning necessary right from the start.

In order to improve the orchard soil, I tried planting several varieties of trees. Among them was the Morishima acacia. This tree grows year round, putting out new buds in all seasons. The aphids which feed on these buds began to multiply in great numbers. Lady bugs fed on the aphids and soon they too began to increase. After the lady bugs had devoured all of the aphids, they climbed down to the citrus trees and started to feed on other insects such as mites, arrowhead scales, and cottony-cushion scales.

Growing fruit without pruning, fertilizing, or using chemical sprays is possible only within a natural environment.

# Orchard Earth

It goes without saying that soil improvement is the fundamental concern of orchard management. If you use chemical fertilizer the trees do grow larger, but year by year the soil becomes depleted. Chemical fertilizer drains the earth of its vitality. If it is used even for one generation the soil suffers considerably.

There is no wiser course in farming than the path of wholesome soil improvement. Twenty years ago, the face of this mountain was bare red clay, so hard you could not stick a shovel into it. A good deal of the land around here was like that. People grew potatoes until the soil was exhausted and then the fields were left abandoned. You might say that, rather than growing citrus and vegetables up here, I have been helping to restore the fertility of the soil.

Let us talk about how I went about restoring those barren mountain slopes. After the war the technique of deeply cultivating a citrus orchard and digging holes for adding organic matter was being encouraged. When I returned from the testing center, I tried doing this in my own orchard. After a few years I came to the conclusion that this method is not only physically exhausting, but, as far as improving the soil is concerned, is just plain useless.

At first I buried straw and ferns which I had brought down from the mountain. Carrying loads of

90 pounds and more was a big job, but after two or three years there was not even enough humus to scoop up in my hand. The trenches I had dug to bury the organic matter caved in and turned into open pits.

Next I tried burying wood. It seems that straw would be the best aid for improving the soil, but judging from the amount of soil formed, wood is better. This is fine as long as there are trees to cut. But for

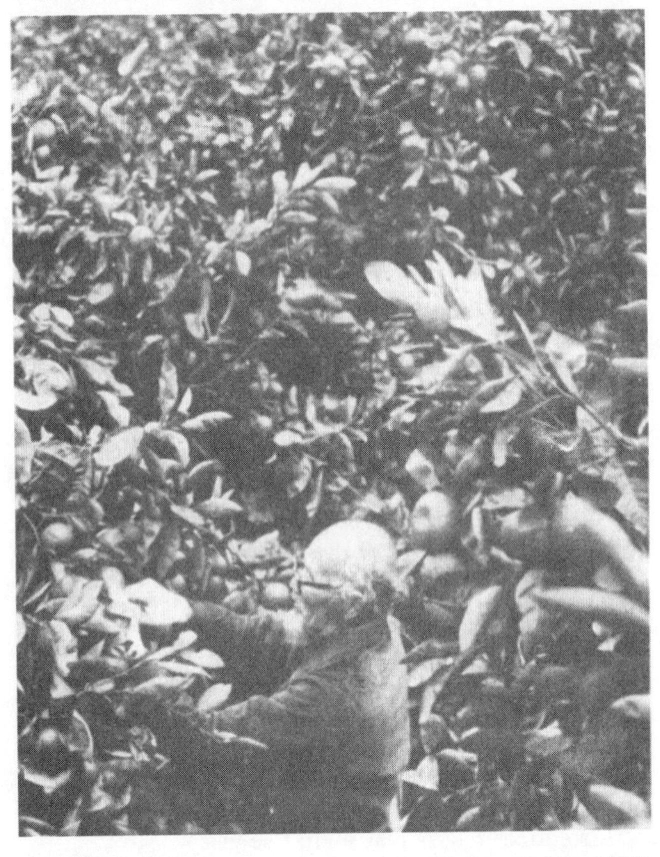

"Twenty years ago the face of this mountain was bare red clay so hard you could not stick a shovel into it."

someone without trees nearby, it is better to grow the wood right in the orchard than to haul it from a distance.

In my orchard there are pines and cedar trees, a few pear trees, persimmons, loquats, Japanese cherries, and many other native varieties growing among the citrus trees. One of the most interesting trees, though not a native, is the Morishima acacia. This is the same tree I mentioned earlier in connection with lady bugs and natural predator protection. The wood is hard, the flowers attract bees, and the leaves are good for fodder. It helps to prevent insect damage in the orchard, acts as a windbreak, and the rhizobium bacteria living within the roots fertilize the soil.

This tree was introduced to Japan from Australia some years ago and grows faster than any tree I have ever seen. It sends out a deep root in just a few months and in six or seven years it stands as tall as a telephone pole. In addition, this tree is a nitrogen fixer, so if 6 to 10 trees are planted to the quarter acre, soil improvement can be carried out in the deep soil strata and there is no need to break your back hauling logs down the mountain.

As for the surface layer of the soil, I sowed a mixture of white clover and alfalfa on the barren ground. It was several years before they could take hold, but finally they came up and covered the orchard hillsides. I also planted Japanese radish (*daikon*). The roots of this hearty vegetable penetrate deeply into the soil, adding organic matter and opening channels for air and water circulation. It reseeds itself easily and after one sowing you can almost forget about it.

As the soil became richer, the weeds started to make a comeback. After seven or eight years, the clover almost disappeared among the weeds, so I tossed out a little more clover seed in late summer after cutting back the weeds.* As a result of this thick weed/clover cover, over the past twenty-five years, the surface layer of the orchard soil, which had been hard red clay, has become loose, dark colored, and rich with earthworms and organic matter.

With the green manure fertilizing the topsoil and the roots of the Morishima acacia improving the soil deep down, you can do quite well without fertilizer and there is no need to cultivate between the orchard trees. With tall trees for windbreaks, citrus in the middle, and a green manure cover below, I have found a way to take it easy and let the orchard manage itself.

---

*During the summer Mr. Fukuoka cuts the weeds, briers, and tree sprouts growing beneath the orchard trees with a scythe.

## Growing Vegetables Like Wild Plants

Next let us talk about growing vegetables. One can either use a backyard garden to supply kitchen vegetables for the household or else grow vegetables on open, unused land.

For the backyard garden it is enough to say that you should grow the right vegetables at the right time in soil prepared by organic compost and manure. The method of growing vegetables for the kitchen table in old Japan blended well with the natural pattern of life. Children play under fruit trees in the backyard. Pigs eat scraps from the kitchen and root around in the soil. Dogs bark and play and the farmer sows seeds in the rich earth. Worms and insects grow up with the vegetables, chickens peck at the worms and lay eggs for the children to eat.

The typical rural family in Japan grew vegetables in this way until not more than twenty years ago.

Plant disease was prevented by growing the traditional crops at the right time, keeping the soil healthy by returning all organic residues to the soil, and rotating crops. Harmful insects were picked off by hand, and also pecked by chickens. In southern Shikoku there was a kind of chicken that would eat worms and insects on the vegetables without scratching the roots or damaging the plants.

Some people may be skeptical at first about using

animal manure and human waste, thinking it primitive or dirty. Today people want "clean" vegetables, so farmers grow them in hothouses without using soil at all. Gravel culture, sand culture, and hydroponics are getting more popular all the time. The vegetables are grown with chemical nutrients and by light which is filtered through a vinyl covering. It is strange that people have come to think of these vegetables grown chemically as "clean" and safe to eat. Foods grown in soil balanced by the action of worms, microorganisms, and decomposing animal manure are the cleanest and most wholesome of all.

In growing vegetables in a "semi-wild" way, making use of a vacant lot, riverbank or open wasteland, my idea is to just toss out the seeds and let the vegetables grow up with the weeds. I grow my vegetables on the mountainside in the spaces between the citrus trees.

The important thing is knowing the right time to plant. For the spring vegetables the right time is when the winter weeds are dying back and just before the summer weeds have sprouted.* For the fall sowing, seeds should be tossed out when the summer grasses are fading away and the winter weeds have not yet appeared.

It is best to wait for a rain which is likely to last

---

*This method of growing vegetables has been developed by Mr. Fukuoka by trial and experiment in accordance with local conditions. Where he lives there are dependable spring rains, and a climate warm enough to grow vegetables in all seasons. Over the years he has come to know which vegetables can be grown among which weeds and the kind of care each requires.

In most parts of North America the specific method Mr. Fukuoka uses for growing vegetables would be impractical. It is up to each farmer who would grow vegetables in the semi-wild manner to develop a technique appropriate to the land and the natural vegetation.

for several days. Cut a swath in the weed cover and put out the vegetable seeds. There is no need to cover them with soil; just lay the weeds you have cut back over the seeds to act as a mulch and to hide them from the birds and chickens until they can germinate. Usually the weeds must be cut back two or three times in order to give the vegetable seedlings a head start, but sometimes just once is enough.

Where the weeds and clover are not so thick, you can simply toss out the seeds. The chickens will eat some of them, but many will germinate. If you plant in a row or furrow, there is a chance that beetles or other insects will devour many of the seeds. They walk in a straight line. Chickens also spot a patch which has been cleared and come to scratch around. It is my experience that it is best to scatter the seeds here and there.

Vegetables grown in this way are stronger than most people think. If they sprout up before the weeds, they will not be overgrown later on. There are some vegetables, such as spinach and carrots, which do not germinate easily. Soaking the seeds in water for a day or two, then wrapping them in a little clay pellet, should solve the problem.

If sown a bit heavily, Japanese radish, turnips, and various leafy green autumn vegetables will be strong enough to compete successfully with the winter and early spring weeds. A few always go unharvested, re-seeding themselves year after year. They have a unique flavor and make very interesting eating.

It is an amazing sight to see many unfamiliar vegetables thriving here and there on the mountain. Japanese radishes and turnips grow half in the soil and half above the surface. Carrots and burdock often grow short and fat with many root hairs, and I believe their tart, slightly bitter flavor is that of their original wild predecessors. Garlic, Japanese pearl onions, and

Chinese leeks, once planted, will come up by themselves year after year.

Legumes are best sown in spring. Cowpeas and kidney beans are easy to grow and give high yields. In growing peas, red *azuki* beans, soy beans, pinto beans, and kidney beans, early germination is essential. They will have difficulty germinating without enough rain, and you must keep an eye out for birds and insects.

Tomatoes and eggplants are not strong enough to compete with the weeds when they are young, and so should be grown in a starter bed and later transplanted. Instead of staking them up, let the tomatoes run along the ground. Roots will grow down from the nodes along the main stem and new shoots will come up and bear fruit.

As for the cucumbers, the creeping-on-the-ground variety is best. You have to take care of the young plants, occasionally cutting the weeds, but after that, the plants will grow strong. Lay out bamboo, or the branches of a tree and the cucumbers will twine all over them. The branches keep the fruit just above the ground so that it does not rot.

This method of growing cucumbers also works for melons and squash.

Potatoes and taros are very strong plants. Once planted they will come up in the same place every year and never be overgrown by weeds. Just leave a few in the ground when you harvest. If the soil is hard, grow Japanese radish first. As their roots grow they cultivate and soften the earth and after a few seasons, potatoes can be grown in their place.

I have found white clover useful in holding back weeds. It grows thickly and can smother out even strong weeds such as mugwort and crabgrass. If the clover is sown mixed with the vegetable seeds, it will act as a living mulch, enriching the soil, and keeping the ground moist and well aerated.

As with vegetables, it is important to choose the right time to sow the clover seed. Late summer or fall sowing is best; the roots develop during the cold months, giving the clover a jump on the annual spring grasses. The clover will also do well if sown early in spring. Either broadcasting or planting in rows about twelve inches apart is fine. Once the clover takes hold, you do not need to sow it again for five or six years.

The main aim of this semi-wild vegetable growing is to grow crops as naturally as possible on land which would otherwise be left unused. If you try to use improved techniques or to get bigger yields the attempt will end in failure. In most cases the failure will be caused by insects or diseases. If various kinds of herbs and vegetables are mixed together and grown among the natural vegetation, damage by insects and diseases will be minimal and there will be no need to use sprays or to pick bugs off by hand.

You can grow vegetables anyplace there is a varied and vigorous growth of weeds. It is important to become familiar with the yearly cycle and growing pattern of the weeds and grasses. By looking at the variety and the size of the weeds in a certain area you can tell what kind of soil is there and whether or not a deficiency exists.

In my orchard I grow burdock, cabbage, tomatoes, carrots, mustard, beans, turnips and many other kinds of herbs and vegetables in this semi-wild way.

# The Terms for Abandoning Chemicals

Today Japanese rice growing stands at an important crossroads. Farmers and specialists are confused as to which path to follow—to continue paddy transplanting, or to move over to direct seeding, and if the latter, to choose cultivation or non-cultivation. I have been saying for the past twenty years that direct seeding non-cultivation will eventually prove to be the best way. The speed with which direct seeding is already spreading in Okayama Prefecture is eye-opening.

There are those, however, who say that turning to a non-chemical agriculture to supply the nation's food is unthinkable. They say that chemical treatments must be used to control the three great rice diseases—stem rot, rice blast disease, and bacterial leaf blight. But if farmers would stop using weak, "improved" seed varieties, stop adding too much nitrogen to the soil, and reduce the amount of irrigation water so that strong roots could develop, these diseases would all but disappear and chemical sprays would become unnecessary.

At first, the red clay soil in my fields was weak and unsuited for growing rice. Brown spot disease frequently occurred. But as the field gradually grew in fertility, the incidence of brown spot disease decreased. Lately there have been no outbreaks at all.

With insect damage the situation is the same. The most important thing is not to kill the natural predators. Keeping the field continuously under water or irrigating with stagnant or polluted water will also lead to insect problems. The most troublesome insect pests, summer and fall leaf-hoppers, can be kept under control by keeping water out of the field.

Green rice leaf-hoppers, living in the weeds over the winter, may become a virus host. If this happens the result is often a loss of ten to twenty percent from rice blast disease. If chemicals are not sprayed, however, there will be many spiders present in the field and one can generally leave the work to them. Spiders are sensitive to even the slightest human tampering and care must always be taken on this account.

Most people think that if chemical fertilizer and insecticides were abandoned agricultural yields would fall to a fraction of the present level. Experts on insect damage estimate that losses in the first year after giving up insecticides would be about five percent. Loss of another five percent in abandoning chemical fertilizer would probably not be far mistaken.

That is, if the use of water in the rice field were curtailed, and the chemical fertilizer and pesticide spraying encouraged by the Agricultural Co-op were abandoned, the average losses in the first year would probably reach about ten percent. The recuperative power of nature is great beyond imagining and after this initial loss, I believe harvests would increase and eventually surpass their original level.

While I was with the Kochi Testing Station, I carried out experiments in the prevention of stem borers. These insects enter and feed on the stem of the rice plant, causing the stalk to turn white and wither. The method of estimating the damage is simple: you count how many white stalks of rice there are. In a hundred plants, ten or twenty percent of the stalks may be white. In severe cases, when it appears as though the whole crop has been ruined, the actual damage is about thirty percent.

To try to avoid this loss, one field of rice was sprayed with insecticide to kill the stem borers; another field was left untreated. When the results were calculated it turned out that the untreated field with many withered stalks had the higher yield. At first I could not believe it myself and thought it was an experimental error. But the data appeared to be accurate, so I investigated further.

What happened was that by attacking the weaker plants the stem borers produced a kind of thinning effect. The withering of some stems left more room for the rest of the plants. Sunlight was then able to penetrate to the lower leaves. These remaining rice plants grew more strongly as a result, sent up more grain-bearing stalks, and produced more grains to the head than they could have without the thinning. When the density of stalks is too great and insects do not thin out the excess, the plants look healthy enough, but in many cases the harvest is actually lower.

Looking at the many research testing center reports you can find the results of using practically every chemical spray on record. But it is generally not realized that only half of these results are reported. Of course there is no intention of hiding anything, but when the results are published by the chemical companies as in advertisements, it is the same as if the conflicting data had been concealed. Results which show lower yields, as in the experiment with the stem borers, are checked off as experimental discrepancies and discarded. There are, of course, cases in which insect extermination results in increased yields, but there are other cases in which the yield is reduced. Reports of the latter rarely appear in print.

Among agricultural chemicals, herbicides are probably the most difficult to dissuade farmers from using. Since ancient times the farmer has been afflicted with what might be termed "the battle against the weeds." Plowing, cultivating between the rows, the ritual of rice transplanting itself, all are mainly aimed at eliminating weeds. Before the development of herbicides, a farmer had to walk many miles through the flooded rice fields each season, pushing a weeding tool up and down the rows and pulling weeds by hand. It is easy to understand why these chemicals were received as a godsend. In the use of straw and clover and the temporary flooding of the fields, I have found a simple way to control weeds without either the hot, hard labor of weeding or the use of chemicals.

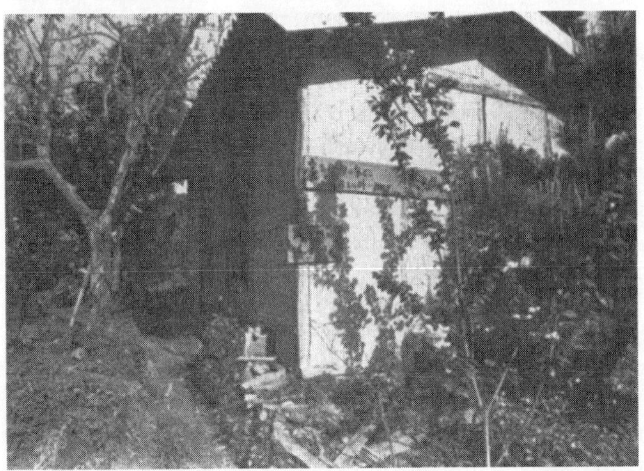

A mudwalled hut in the orchard.

## Limits of the Scientific Method

Before researchers become researchers they should become philosophers. They should consider what the human goal is, what it is that humanity should create. Doctors should first determine at the fundamental level what it is that human beings depend on for life.

In applying my theories to farming, I have been experimenting in growing my crops in various ways, always with the idea of developing a method close to nature. I have done this by whittling away unnecessary agricultural practices.

Modern scientific agriculture, on the other hand, has no such vision. Research wanders about aimlessly, each researcher seeing just one part of the infinite array of natural factors which affect harvest yields. Furthermore, these natural factors change from place to place and from year to year.

Even though it is the same quarter acre, the farmer must grow his crops differently each year in accordance with variations in weather, insect populations, the condition of the soil, and many other natural factors. Nature is everywhere in perpetual motion; conditions are never exactly the same in any two years.

Modern research divides nature into tiny pieces and conducts tests that conform neither with natural law nor with practical experiences. The results are arranged for the convenience of research, not according to the needs of the farmer. To think that these conclusions can be put to use with invariable success in the farmer's field is a big mistake.

Recently Professor Tsuno of Ehime University wrote a lengthy book on the relationship of plant metabolism to rice harvests. This professor often comes to my field, digs down a few feet to check the soil, brings students along to measure the angle of sunlight and shade and whatnot, and takes plant specimens back to the lab for analysis. I often ask him, "When you go back, are you going to try non-cultivation direct seeding?" He laughingly answers, "No, I'll leave the applications to you. I'm going to stick to research."

So that is how it is. You study the function of the plant's metabolism and its ability to absorb nutrients from the soil, write a book, and get a doctorate in agricultural science. But do not ask if your theory of assimilation is going to be relevant to the yield.

Even if you can explain how metabolism affects the productivity of the top leaf when the average temperature is eighty-four degrees (Fahrenheit), there are places where the temperature is not eighty-four degrees. And if the temperature is eighty-four degrees in Ehime this year, next year it may only be seventy-five degrees. To say that simply stepping up metabolism will increase starch formation and produce a large harvest is a mistake. The geography and topography of the land, the condition of the soil, its structure, texture, and drainage, exposure to sunlight, insect relationships, the variety of seed used, the method of cultivation—truly an infinite variety of factors—must all be considered. A scientific testing method which takes all relevant factors into account is an impossibility.

You hear a lot of talk these days about the benefits of the "Good Rice Movement" and the "Green Revolution." Because these methods depend on weak, "improved" seed varieties, it becomes necessary for the farmer to apply chemicals and insecticides eight or ten times during the growing season. In a short time the soil is burned clean of microorganisms and organic matter. The life of the soil is destroyed and crops come to be dependent on nutrients added from the outside in the form of chemical fertilizer.

It appears that things go better when the farmer applies "scientific" techniques, but this does not mean that science must come to the rescue because the natural fertility is inherently insufficient. It means that rescue is necessary because the natural fertility has been destroyed.

By spreading straw, growing clover, and returning to the soil all organic residues, the earth comes to possess all the nutrients needed to grow rice and winter grain in the same field year after year. By natural farming, fields that have already been damaged by cultivation or the use of agricultural chemicals can be effectively rehabilitated.

# III

# One Farmer Speaks Out

There is a great deal of concern in Japan these days, and justifiably so, about the deteriorating quality of the environment and the resulting contamination of food. Citizens have organized boycotts and large demonstrations to protest the indifference of political and industrial leaders. But all of this activity, if carried out in the present spirit, only results in wasted effort. To talk about cleaning up specific cases of pollution is like treating symptoms of a disease while the root cause of the malady continues to fester.

Two years ago, for instance, a conference for the purpose of discussing pollution was organized by the Agricultural Management Research Center, together with the Organic Agricultural Council and the Nada Co-op. The chairman of the conference was Mr. Teruo Ichiraku, who is head of the Japanese Organic Farmers Association, and is also one of the most powerful figures in the government's Agricultural Co-op. The recommendations of this agency as to which crops and seed varieties should be grown, how much fertilizer should be used and which chemicals should be applied are followed by nearly every village farmer in Japan.

Because such a diversity of influential people were taking part, I attended with hopes that far-reaching action could be decided upon and put into effect.

From the standpoint of publicizing the food pollution problem, this conference could be said to have been successful. But like the other meetings, the discussions degenerated into a series of highly technical reports by research specialists and personal accounts of the horrors of food contamination. No one seemed willing to address the problem at its fundamental level.

In a discussion of mercury poisoning of tuna, for example, the representative of the Fisheries Bureau first spoke of how truly frightening the problem had become. At that time mercury pollution was being discussed every day on the radio and in the newspapers, and so everyone listened closely to hear what he had to say.

The speaker said that the amount of mercury in the bodies of tuna, even those taken in the Antarctic Ocean and near the North Pole, was extremely high. However, when a laboratory specimen taken several hundred years ago was dissected and analyzed, this fish, contrary to expectation, also contained mercury. His tentative conclusion suggested that mercury consumption was necessary for the fish to live.

The people in the audience looked at each other in disbelief. The purpose of the meeting was supposed to have been to determine how to deal with the pollution which had already contaminated the environment, and to take measures to correct it. Instead, here was this representative from the Fisheries Bureau saying that mercury is necessary for the tuna's survival. This is what I mean when I say that people do not grasp the root cause of pollution but only see it from a narrow and superficial perspective.

I stood up and suggested that we take joint action to set up, then and there, a concrete plan to deal with pollution. Would it not be better to talk straightforwardly about discontinuing the use of the chemicals which are causing the pollution? Rice, for example can be grown very well without chemicals, as can citrus, and it is not difficult to grow vegetables that way either. I said that it could be done, and that I had been doing it on my farm for years, but that as long as the government continued to endorse the use of chemicals, no one else would give clean farming a try.

Members of the Fisheries Bureau were present at the meeting, as were people from the Ministry of Agriculture and Forestry and the Agricultural Co-op. If they and the chairman of the conference, Mr. Ichiraku, had really wanted to get things going and had suggested that farmers throughout the country should try growing rice without chemicals, sweeping changes could have been made.

There was one great problem, however. If crops were to be grown without agricultural chemicals, fertilizer, or machinery, the giant chemical companies would become unnecessary and the government's Agricultural Co-op Agency would collapse. To put the matter right out front, I said that the Co-ops and the modern agricultural policy-makers depend on large capital investment in fertilizer and agricultural machinery for their base of power. To do away with machinery and chemicals would bring about a complete change in the economic and social structures. Therefore, I could see no way that Mr. Ichiraku, the Co-ops or the government officials could speak out in favor of measures to clean up pollution.

When I spoke out in this way, the chairman said, "Mr. Fukuoka, you are upsetting the conference with your remarks," shutting my mouth for me. Well, that's what happened.

# A Modest Solution to a Difficult Problem

So it appears that government agencies have no intention of stopping pollution. A second difficulty is that all aspects of the problem of food pollution must be brought together and solved at the same time. A problem cannot be solved by people who are concerned with only one or another of its parts.

To the extent that the consciousness of everyone is not fundamentally transformed, pollution will not cease.

For example, the farmer thinks that the Inland Sea* is of no concern to him. He thinks that it is the officials of the Fisheries Bureau whose business it is to look after fish, and that it is the job of the Environmental Council to take care of ocean pollution. In this way of thinking lies the problem.

The most commonly used chemical fertilizers, ammonium sulfate, urea, super phosphate and the like, are used in large amounts, only fractions of which are absorbed by the plants in the field. The rest leaches into streams and rivers, eventually flowing into the Inland Sea. These nitrogen compounds become food for algae and plankton which multiply in great numbers, causing the red tide to appear. Of

*The small sea between the islands of Honshu, Kyushu and Shikoku.

course, industrial discharge of mercury and other contaminating wastes also contribute to the pollution, but for the most part water pollution in Japan comes from agricultural chemicals.

So it is the farmer who must shoulder major responsibility for the red tide. The farmer who applies polluting chemicals to his field, the corporations who manufacture these chemicals, the village officials who believe in the convenience of chemicals and offer technical guidance accordingly—if each of these people does not ponder the problem deeply there will be no solving the question of water pollution.

As it is now, only those who are most directly affected become active in trying to cope with pollution problems, as in the case of the local fishermen's struggle against the big oil companies after the oil spill near Mizushima. Or else some professor proposes to cope with the problem by opening a channel through the belly of Shikoku Island to let the relatively clean water of the Pacific Ocean flow into the Inland Sea. This sort of thing is researched and attempted time after time, but a true solution can never come about in this way.

The fact of the matter is that whatever we do, the situation gets worse. The more elaborate the countermeasures, the more complicated the problems become.

Suppose a pipe *were* laid across Shikoku and water *were* pumped up from the Pacific and poured into the Inland Sea. Let us say that this may possibly clean up the Inland Sea. But where is the electric power going to come from to run the factory which will manufacture the steel pipe, and how about the power required to pump the water up? A nuclear power plant would become necessary. To construct such a system, concrete and all the various materials must be assembled, and a uranium processing center built as well. When solutions develop in this way, they only sow the seeds for second- and third-generation pollution problems which will be more difficult than the previous ones, and more widespread.

It is like the case of the greedy farmer who opens the irrigation inlet too wide and lets the water come rushing into his rice paddy. A crack develops and the ridge crumbles away. At this point reinforcement work becomes necessary. The walls are strengthened and the irrigation channel enlarged. The increased volume of water only increases the potential danger, and the next time the ridge weakens, even greater effort will be required for reconstruction.

When a decision is made to cope with the symptoms of a problem, it is generally assumed that the corrective measures will solve the problem itself. They seldom do. Engineers cannot seem to get this through their heads. These countermeasures are all based on too narrow a definition of what is wrong. Human measures and countermeasures proceed from limited scientific truth and judgment. A true solution can never come about in this way.*

My modest solutions, such as spreading straw and growing clover, create no pollution. They are effective because they eliminate the source of the problem. Until the modern faith in big technological solutions can be overturned, pollution will only get worse.

---

*By "limited scientific truth and judgment," Mr. Fukuoka is referring to the world as perceived and constructed by the human intellect. He considers this perception to be limited to a framework defined by its own assumptions.

# The Fruit of Hard Times

Consumers generally assume that they have nothing to do with causing agricultural pollution. Many of them ask for food that has not been chemically treated. But chemically treated food is marketed mainly in response to the preferences of the consumer. The consumer demands large, shiny, unblemished produce of regular shape. To satisfy these desires, agricultural chemicals which were not used five or six years ago have come rapidly into use.

How did we get into such a predicament? People say they do not care if cucumbers are straight or crooked, and that fruit does not necessarily have to be beautiful on the outside. But take a look inside the wholesale markets in Tokyo sometime if you want to see how the price responds to consumer preferences. When the fruit looks just a little better, you get a premium of five or ten cents a pound. When the fruit is classed "Small," "Medium" or "Large," the price per pound may double or triple with each increase in size.

The consumer's willingness to pay high prices for food produced out of season has also contributed to the increased use of artificial growing methods and chemicals. Last year, Unshu mandarin oranges grown in hothouses for summer shipment* fetched prices

*This fruit ripens naturally late in the fall.

ten to twenty times higher than seasonal mandarins. Instead of the usual price of 10 to 15 cents per pound, outrageous prices of $.80, $1.00, even $1.75 to the pound were paid. And so, if you invest several thousand dollars to install the equipment, buy the necessary fuel, and work the extra hours, you can realize a profit.

Farming out of season is becoming more and more popular all the time. To have mandarin oranges just one month earlier, the people in the city seem happy enough to pay for the farmer's extra investment in labor and equipment. But if you ask how important it is for human beings to have this fruit a month earlier, the truth is that it is not important at all, and money is not the only price paid for such indulgence.

Furthermore, a coloring agent, not used a few years ago, is now being used. With this chemical, the fruit becomes fully colored one week earlier. Depending on whether the fruit is sold a week before or after the 10th of October, the price either doubles or falls by half, so the farmer applies color-accelerating chemicals, and after the harvest places the fruit in a ripening room for gas treatment.

But when the fruit is shipped out early, it is not sweet enough, and so artificial sweeteners are used. It is generally thought that chemical sweeteners have been prohibited, but the artificial sweetener sprayed on citrus trees has not been specifically outlawed. The question is whether or not it falls into the category of "agricultural chemicals." In any case, almost everybody is using it.

The fruit is then taken to the co-op fruit-sorting center. In order to separate the fruit into large and small sizes, each one is sent rolling several hundred yards down a long conveyor. Bruising is common. The larger the sorting center, the longer the fruit is bounced and tumbled about. After a water washing the mandarin oranges are sprayed with preservatives and a coloring agent is brushed on. Finally, as a finishing touch, a paraffin wax solution is applied and the fruit is polished to a glossy shine. Nowadays fruit is really "run through the mill."

So from the time just before the fruit has been harvested to the time it is shipped out and put on the display counter, five or six chemicals are used. This is not to mention the chemical fertilizers and sprays that were used while the crops were growing in the orchard. And this is all because the consumer wants to buy fruit just a little more attractive. This little edge of preference has put the farmer in a real predicament.

These measures are not taken because the farmer likes to work this way, or because the officials of the Ministry of Agriculture enjoy putting the farmer through all this extra labor, but until the general sense of values changes, the situation will not improve.

When I was with the Yokohama Customs Office forty years ago, Sunkist lemons and oranges were being handled in this way. I was strongly opposed to introducing this system to Japan, but my words could not prevent the current system from being adopted.

If one farm household or co-op takes up a new process such as the waxing of mandarin oranges, because of the extra care and attention the profit is higher. The other agricultural co-ops take notice and soon they, too, adopt the new process. Fruit which is not wax-treated no longer brings so high a price. In two or three years waxing is taken up all over the country. The competition then brings the prices down, and all that is left to the farmer is the burden of hard work and the added costs of supplies and equipment. Now he *must* apply the wax.

Of course the consumer suffers as a result. Food

that is not fresh can be sold because it *looks* fresh. Speaking biologically, fruit in a slightly shriveled state is holding its respiration and energy consumption down to the lowest possible level. It is like a person in meditation: his metabolism, respiration, and calorie consumption reach an extremely low level. Even if he fasts, the energy within the body will be conserved. In the same way, when mandarin oranges grow wrinkled, when fruit shrivels, when vegetables wilt, they are in the state that will preserve their food value for the longest possible time.

It is a mistake to try to maintain the mere appearance of freshness, as when shopkeepers sprinkle water on their vegetables over and over again. Although the vegetables are kept looking fresh, their flavor and nutritional value soon deteriorate.

At any rate, all the agricultural cooperatives and collective sorting centers have been integrated and expanded to carry out such unnecessary activities. This is called "modernization." The produce is packed and loaded onto the great delivery system and shipped off to the consumer.

To say it in a word, until there is a reversal of the sense of values which cares more for size and appearance than for quality, there will be no solving the problem of food pollution.

## The Marketing of Natural Food

For the past several years I have sent 88 to 110 bushels (5,000-6,500 pounds) of rice to natural food stores in various parts of the country. I have also shipped 400 thirty-five-pound cartons of mandarin oranges in ten-ton trucks to the co-op living association in Tokyo's Suginami district. The chairman of the co-op wanted to sell unpolluted produce, and this formed the basis of our agreement.

The first year was quite successful but there were also some complaints. The size of the fruit was too varied, the exterior was a bit dirty, the skin was sometimes shriveled and so on. I had shipped the fruit in plain unmarked cartons, and there were some people who suspected, without reason, that the fruit was just an assortment of "seconds." I now pack the fruit in cartons lettered "natural mandarins."

Since natural food can be produced with the least expense and effort, I reason that it should be sold at the cheapest price. Last year, in the Tokyo area, my fruit was the lowest priced of all. According to many shopkeepers the flavor was the most delicious. It would be best, of course, if the fruit could be sold locally, eliminating the time and expense involved in shipping, but even so, the price was right, the fruit was free of chemicals and it tasted good. This year I have been asked to ship two or three times as much as before.

At this point the question arises as to how far the direct sale of natural food can spread. I have one hope in this regard. Lately chemical fruit growers have been driven into an extremely tight economic pinch, and this makes the production of natural food more attractive to them. No matter how hard the average farmer works applying chemicals, coloring, waxing, and so on, he can only sell his fruit for a price that will barely cover expenses. This year, even a farm with exceptionally fine fruit can only expect to realize a profit of less than five cents per pound. The farmer producing slightly lower quality fruit will end up with nothing at all.

Since prices have slumped in the past few years, the agricultural co-ops and sorting centers have become very strict, selecting fruit of only the very highest quality. Inferior fruit cannot be sold to the sorting centers. After putting in a full day's work in the orchard harvesting the mandarin oranges, loading them into boxes, and carrying them to the sorting shed, the farmer must work until eleven or twelve o'clock at night, picking over his fruit, one by one, keeping only those of perfect size and shape.*

The "good ones" sometimes average only 25% to 50% of the total crop, and even some of these are rejected by the co-op. If the profit remaining is a mere two or three cents per pound, it is considered pretty good. The poor citrus farmer is working hard these days and still barely breaking even.

Growing fruit without applying chemicals, using fertilizer, or cultivating the soil involves less expense, and the farmer's net profit is therefore higher. The fruit I ship out is practically unsorted; I just pack the fruit into a box, send them off to the market, and get to bed early.

---

*The rejected fruit is sold for about half price to a private company to be squeezed for juice.

The other farmers in my neighborhood realize that they are working very hard only to end up with nothing in their pockets. The feeling is growing that there is nothing strange about growing natural food products, and the producers are ready for a change to farming without chemicals. But until natural food can be distributed locally, the average farmer will worry about not having a market in which to sell his produce.

As for the consumer, the common belief has been that natural food should be expensive. If it is not expensive, people suspect that it is not natural food. One retailer remarked to me that no one would buy natural produce unless it is priced high.

I still feel that natural food should be sold more cheaply than any other. Several years ago I was asked to send the honey gathered in the citrus orchard and the eggs laid by the hens on the mountain to a natural food store in Tokyo. When I found out that the merchant was selling them at extravagant prices, I was furious. I knew that a merchant who would take advantage of his customers in that way would also mix my rice with other rice to increase the weight, and that it, too, would reach the consumer at an unfair price. I immediately stopped all shipments to that store.

If a high price is charged for natural food, it means that the merchant is taking excessive profits. Furthermore, if natural foods are expensive, they become luxury foods and only rich people are able to afford them.

If natural food is to become widely popular, it must be available locally at a reasonable price. If the consumer will only adjust to the idea that low prices do not mean that the food is not natural, then everyone will begin thinking in the right direction.

## Commercial Agriculture Will Fail

When the concept of commercial agriculture first appeared, I opposed it. Commercial agriculture in Japan is not profitable for the farmer. Among merchants the rule is that if an article which originally costs a certain amount is further processed, an extra cost is added when the article is sold. But in Japanese agriculture it is not so straightforward. Fertilizer, feed, equipment, and chemicals are purchased at prices fixed abroad, and there is no telling what the actual cost per pound will be when these imported products are used. It is completely up to the merchants. And with selling prices also fixed, the farmer's income is at the mercy of forces beyond his control.

In general, commercial agriculture is an unstable proposition. The farmer would do much better by growing the food he needs without thinking about making money. If you plant one grain of rice, it becomes more than one thousand grains. One row of turnips makes enough pickles for the entire winter. If you follow this line of thought, you will have enough to eat, more than enough, without struggling. But if you decide to try to make money instead, you get on board the profit wagon, and it runs away with you.

I have been thinking lately about white leghorns. Because the improved variety of white leghorn lays over 200 days a year, raising them for profit is considered good business. When raised commercially these chickens are cooped up in long rows of small cages not unlike cells in a penitentiary, and through their entire lives their feet are never allowed to touch the ground. Disease is common and the birds are pumped full of antibiotics and fed a formula diet of vitamins and hormones.

It is said that the local chickens that have been kept since ancient times, the brown and black *shamo* and *chabo*, have only half the egg-laying capacity. As a result these birds have all but disappeared in Japan. I let two hens and one rooster loose to run wild on the mountainside and after one year there were twenty-four. When it seemed that few eggs were being laid, the local birds were busy raising chickens.

In the first year, the leghorn has a greater egg-laying efficiency than the local chickens, but after one year the white leghorn is exhausted and cast aside, whereas the *shamo* we started with has become ten healthy birds running about beneath the orchard

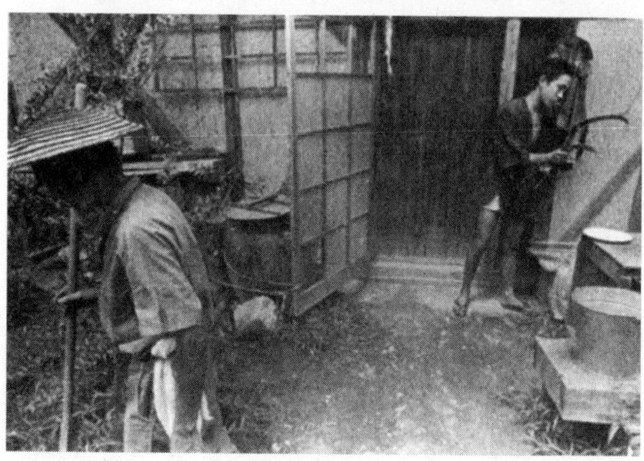

Setting out for a day's work.

trees. Furthermore, the white leghorns lay well because they are raised on artificially enriched feed which is imported from foreign countries and must be bought from the merchants. The local birds scratch around and feed freely on seeds and insects in the area and lay delicious, natural eggs.

If you think commercial vegetables are nature's own, you are in for a big surprise. These vegetables are a watery chemical concoction of nitrogen, phosphorous, and potash, with a little help from the seed. And that is just how they taste. And commercial chicken eggs (you can call them eggs if you like) are nothing more than a mixture of synthetic feed, chemicals, and hormones. This is not a product of nature but a man made synthetic in the shape of an egg. The farmer who produces vegetables and eggs of this kind, I call a manufacturer.

Now if it is manufacturing you are talking about, you will have to do some fancy figuring if you want to make a profit. Since the commercial farmer is not making any money, he is like a merchant who cannot handle the abacus. That sort of fellow is regarded as a fool by other people and his profits are soaked up by politicians and salesmen.

In olden times there were warriors, farmers, craftsmen, and merchants. Agriculture was said to be closer to the source of things than trade or manufacturing, and the farmer was said to be "the cupbearer of the gods." He was always able to get by somehow or other and have enough to eat.

But now there is all this commotion about making money. Ultra-fashionable produce such as grapes, tomatoes, and melons are being grown. Flowers and fruit are being produced out-of-season in hothouses. Fish breeding has been introduced and cattle are raised because profits are high.

This pattern shows clearly what happens when

farming climbs aboard the economic roller coaster. Fluctuations in prices are violent. There are profits, but there are losses as well.

Failure is inevitable. Japanese agriculture has lost sight of its direction and has become unstable. It has strayed away from the basic principles of agriculture and has become a business.

## Research for Whose Benefit?

When I first began direct-seeding rice and winter grain, I was planning to harvest with a hand sickle and so I thought it would be more convenient to set the seeds out in regular rows. After many attempts, dabbling about as an amateur, I produced a handmade seeding tool. Thinking that this tool might be of practical use to other farmers, I brought it to the man at the testing center. He told me that since we were in an age of large-sized machinery he could not be bothered with my "contraption."

Next I went to a manufacturer of agricultural equipment. I was told here that such a simple machine, no matter how much you tried to make of it, could not be sold for more than $3.50 apiece. "If we made a gadget like that, the farmers might start thinking they didn't need the tractors we sell for thousands of dollars." He said that nowadays the idea is to invent rice planting machines quickly, sell them head over heels for as long as possible, then introduce something newer. Instead of small tractors, they wanted to change over to larger-sized models, and my device was, to them, a step backward. To meet the demands of the times, resources are poured into furthering useless research, and to this day my patent remains on the shelf.

It is the same with fertilizer and chemicals. Instead of developing fertilizer with the farmer in mind, the emphasis is on developing something new, anything at all, in order to make money. After the technicians leave their jobs at the testing centers, they move right over to work for the large chemical companies.

Recently I was talking with Mr. Asada, a technical official in the Ministry of Agriculture and Forestry, and he told me an interesting story. The vegetables grown in hothouses are extremely unsavory. Hearing that the eggplants shipped out in winter have no vitamins and the cucumbers no flavor, he researched the matter and found the reason: certain of the sun's rays could not penetrate the vinyl and glass enclosures in which the vegetables were being grown. His investigation moved over to the lighting system inside the hothouses.

The fundamental question here is whether or not it is necessary for human beings to eat eggplants and cucumbers during the winter. But, this point aside, the only reason they are grown during the winter is that they can be sold then at a good price. Somebody develops a means to grow them, and after some time passes, it is found that these vegetables have no nutritional value. Next, the technician thinks that if the nutrients are being lost, a way must be found to prevent that loss. Because the trouble is thought to be with the lighting system, he begins to research light rays. He thinks everything will be all right if he can produce a hothouse eggplant with vitamins in it. I was told that there are some technicians who devote their entire lives to this kind of research.

Naturally, since such great efforts and resources have gone into producing this eggplant, and the vegetable is said to be high in nutritional value, it is tagged at an even higher price and sells well. "If it is profitable, and if you can sell it, there can't be anything wrong with it."

No matter how hard people try, they cannot improve upon naturally grown fruits and vegetables. Produce grown in an unnatural way satisfies people's fleeting desires but weakens the human body and alters the body chemistry so that it is dependent upon such foods. When this happens, vitamin supplements and medicines become necessary. This situation only creates hardships for the farmer and suffering for the consumer.

# What is Human Food?

The other day someone from NHK television came by and asked me to say something about the flavor of natural food. We talked, and then I asked him to compare the eggs laid by the hens in the coop down below with those of the chickens running free up in the orchard. He found that the yolks of the eggs laid by the chickens cooped up on the typical chicken ranch were soft and watery and their color was pale yellow. He observed that the yolks of the eggs laid by the chickens living wild on the mountain were firm and resilient and bright orange in color. When the old man who runs the *sushi* restaurant in town tasted one of these natural eggs, he said that this was a "real egg," just like in the old days, and rejoiced as if it were some precious treasure.

Again, up in the tangerine orchard, there are many different vegetables growing among the weeds and clover. Turnips, burdock, cucumbers and squash, peanuts, carrots, edible chrysanthemums, potatoes, onions, leaf mustard, cabbage, several varieties of beans, and many other herbs and vegetables are all growing together. The conversation turned to whether or not these vegetables, which had been grown in a semi-wild manner, had a better flavor than those grown in the home garden or with the aid of chemical fertilizer in the fields. When we compared them, the taste was completely different, and we determined that the "wild" vegetables possessed a richer flavor.

I told the reporter that when vegetables are grown in a prepared field using chemical fertilizer, nitrogen, phosphorus and potash are supplied. But when vegetables are grown with natural ground cover in soil naturally rich in organic matter, they get a more balanced diet of nutrients. A great variety of weeds and grasses means that a variety of essential nutrients and micronutrients are available to the vegetables. Plants which grow in such balanced soil have a more subtle flavor.

Edible herbs and wild vegetables, plants growing on the mountain and in the meadow, are very high in nutritional value and are also useful as medicine. Food and medicine are not two different things: they are the front and back of one body. Chemically grown vegetables may be eaten for food, but they cannot be used as medicine.

When you gather and eat the seven herbs of spring,* your spirit becomes gentle. And when you eat bracken shoots, osmund and shepherd's purse, you become calm. To calm restless, impatient feelings, shepherd's purse is the best of all. They say that if children eat shepherd's purse, willow buds or insects living in trees, this will cure violent crying tantrums, and in the old days children were often made to eat them. *Daikon* (Japanese radish) has for its ancestor the plant called *nazuna* (shepherd's purse), and this word *nazuna* is related to the word *nagomu,* which means to be softened. *Daikon* is the "herb that softens one's disposition."

Among wild foods insects are often overlooked.

---

*Watercress, shepherd's purse, wild turnip, cottonweed, chickweed, wild radish, and bee nettle. Illustrated on pg. 121.

During the war, when I worked at the research center, I was assigned to determine what insects in Southeast Asia could be eaten. When I investigated this matter, I was amazed to discover that almost any insect is edible.

For example, no one would think that lice or fleas could be of any use at all, but lice, ground up and eaten with winter grain, are a remedy for epilepsy, and fleas are a medicine for frostbite. All insect larvae are quite edible, but they must be alive. Poring over the old texts, I found stories having to do with "delicacies" prepared from maggots from the outhouse, and the flavor of the familiar silkworm was said to be

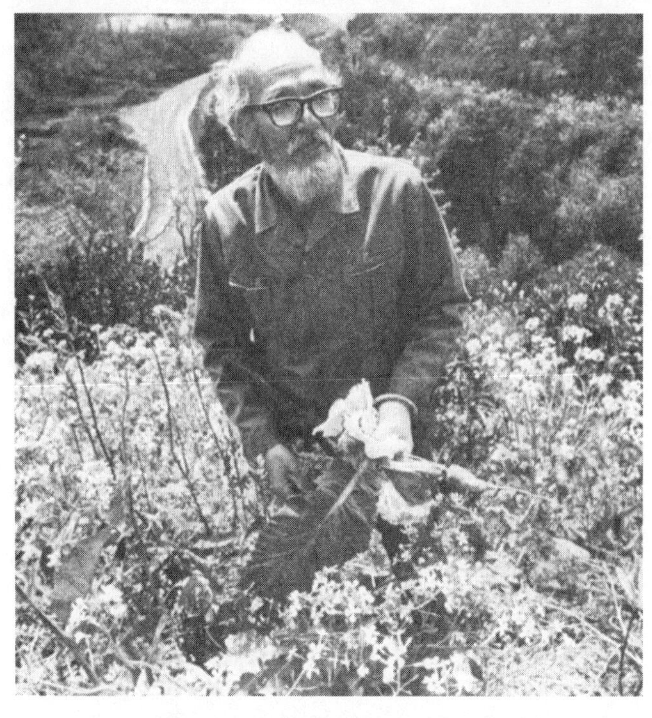

In a patch of mustard and wild turnips.

exquisite beyond compare. Even moths, if you shake the powder off their wings first, are very tasty.

So, whether from the standpoint of flavor or from the standpoint of health, many things which people consider repulsive are actually quite tasty and also good for the human body.

Vegetables that are biologically closest to their wild ancestors are the best in flavor and the highest in food value. For example, in the lily family (which includes *nira*, garlic, Chinese leek, green onion, pearl onion, and bulb onion) the *nira* and Chinese leek are highest in nutrition, good as herbal medicine, and also useful as a tonic for general well-being. To most people, however, the more domestic varieties, such as green onion and bulb onion, are regarded as the best tasting. For some reason, modern people like the flavor of vegetables that have departed from their wild state.

A similar taste preference applies to animal foods. Wild birds when eaten, are much better for the body than domestic fowl such as chickens and ducks, and yet these birds, raised in an environment far removed from their natural homes, are regarded as good tasting and sold at high prices. Goat's milk has a higher food value than cow's milk, but it is the cow's milk which is in greater demand.

Foods that have departed far from their wild state and those raised chemically or in a completely contrived environment unbalance the body chemistry. The more out of balance one's body becomes, the more one comes to desire unnatural foods. This situation is dangerous to health.

To say that what one eats is merely a matter of preference is deceiving, because an unnatural or exotic diet creates a hardship for the farmer and the fisherman as well. It seems to me that the greater one's desires, the more one has to work to satisfy them. Some fish, such as the popular tuna and yellowtail must be caught in distant waters, but sardine, sea bream, flounder, and other small fish can be caught in great abundance in the Inland Sea. Speaking nutritionally, creatures which live in freshwater rivers and streams, such as carp, pond snails, stream crayfish, marsh crabs and so on, are better for the body than those from salt water. Next come shallow-water ocean fish, and finally fish from deep salt water and from distant seas. The foods that are nearby are best for human beings, and things that he has to struggle to obtain turn out to be the least beneficial of all.

That is to say that if one accepts what is near at hand, all goes well. If the farmers who live in this village eat only the foods that can be grown or gathered here, there will be no mistake. In the end, like the group of young people living in the huts up in the orchard, one will find it simplest to eat brown rice and unpolished barley, millet, and buckwheat, together with the seasonal plants and semi-wild vegetables. One ends up with the best food; it has flavor, and is good for the body.

If 22 bushels (1,300 pounds) of rice and 22 bushels of winter grain are harvested from a quarter acre field such as one of these, then the field will support five to ten people each investing an average of less than one hour of labor per day. But if the field were turned over to pasturage, or if the grain were fed to cattle, only one person could be supported per quarter acre. Meat becomes a luxury food when its production requires land which could provide food directly for human consumption.* This has been shown clearly and defi-

*Although most meat in North America is produced by feeding field crops such as wheat, barley, corn, and soybeans to animals, there are also large areas of land best used when rotated regularly into pasture or hayfields. In Japan, almost no such land exists. Almost all meat must be imported.

nitely. Each person should ponder seriously how much hardship he is causing by indulging in food so expensively produced.

Meat and other imported foods are luxuries because they require more energy and resources than the traditional vegetables and grains produced locally. It follows that people who limit themselves to a simple local diet need do less work and use less land than those with an appetite for luxury.

If people continue to eat meat and imported food, within ten years it is certain that Japan will fall into a food crisis. Within thirty years, there will be overwhelming shortages. The absurd idea has swept in from somewhere that a change from rice-eating to bread-eating indicates an improvement in the everyday life of the Japanese people. Actually this is not so. Brown rice and vegetables may seem to be coarse fare, but this is the very finest diet nutritionally, and enables human beings to live simply and directly.

If we do have a food crisis it will not be caused by the insufficiency of nature's productive power, but by the extravagance of human desire.

# A Merciful Death for Barley

Forty years ago, as a result of increasing political hostility between the United States and Japan, importing wheat from America became impossible. There was a general movement throughout the country to grow wheat domestically. The American wheat varieties being used require a long growing season and the grain finally matured in the middle of Japan's rainy season. Even after the farmer had taken such great pains to grow the crop, it would often rot during the harvest. These varieties proved to be very unreliable and highly susceptible to disease, so the farmers did not want to grow wheat. When ground and toasted in the traditional way, the taste was so terrible that you almost choked and had to spit it out.

The traditional varieties of Japanese rye and barley can be harvested in May, before the rainy season, so they are comparatively safe crops. Farmers had wheat cultivation forced upon them nonetheless. Everyone laughed and said there was nothing worse than growing wheat, but they patiently went along with the government policy.

After the war, American wheat was again imported in large quantities, causing the price of wheat grown in Japan to fall. This added to the many other good reasons to discontinue wheat growing. "Give up wheat, give up wheat!" was the slogan propagated nationwide by the government's agricultural leaders, and the farmers gladly gave it up. At the same time, because of the low price of imported wheat, the government encouraged the farmers to stop growing the traditional winter crops of rye and barley. This policy was carried out and the fields of Japan were left to lie fallow through the winter.

About ten years ago I was chosen to represent Ehime Prefecture in NHK television's "Outstanding Farmer of the Year" competition. At that time I was asked by a member of the screening committee, "Mr. Fukuoka, why don't you give up growing rye and barley?" I answered, "Rye and barley are easy crops to raise, and by growing them in succession with rice we can produce the greatest number of calories from Japan's fields. That's why I don't give them up."

It was made clear that no one who stubbornly goes against the will of the Ministry of Agriculture could be named Outstanding Farmer and I then said, "If that's what keeps someone from getting the Outstanding Farmer Award, then I'm better off without it." One of the members of the screening panel later said to me, "If I were to leave the university and take up farming myself, I would probably farm as you do, and grow rice in summer, and barley and rye over the winter every year as before the war."

Shortly after this episode, I appeared on an NHK television program in a panel discussion with various university professors, and at that time I was again asked, "Why don't you give up growing rye and barley?" I stated once again, very clearly, that I wasn't about to give them up for any one of a dozen good reasons. About that time the slogan for giving up winter grain cultivation called for "A merciful death." That is, the practice of growing winter grain and rice in succession should pass away quietly. But "merciful death" is too gentle a term; the Ministry of

Agriculture really wanted it to die in the ditch. When it became clear to me that the main purpose of the program was to promote a rapid end to growing winter grain, leaving it "dead by the side of the road" so to speak, I exploded in indignation.

Forty years ago the call was to grow wheat, to grow foreign grain, to grow a useless and impossible crop. Then it was said that the Japanese varieties of rye and barley did not have as high a food value as American grain and the farmers regretfully gave up growing these traditional grains. As the standard of living rose by leaps and bounds, the word went out to eat meat, eat eggs, drink milk, and change from eating rice to eating bread. Corn, soybeans, and wheat were imported in ever-increasing quantities. American wheat was cheap, so the growing of native rye and barley was abandoned. Japanese agriculture adopted measures which forced farmers to take part-time jobs in town so they could buy the crops they had been told not to grow.

And now, new concern has arisen over the shortage of food resources. Self-sufficiency in rye and bar-

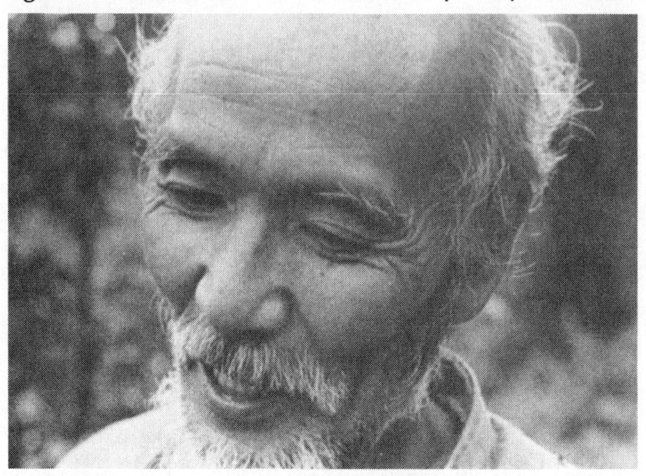

ley production is again being advocated. They are saying there will even be subsidies. But it is not enough to grow traditional winter grains for a couple of years and then to abandon them again. A sound agricultural policy must be established. Because the Ministry of Agriculture has no clear idea of what should be grown in the first place, and because it does not understand the connection between what is grown in the fields and the people's diet, a consistent agricultural policy remains an impossibility.

If the Ministry's staff were to go to the mountains and meadows, gather the seven herbs of spring, and the seven herbs of autumn,* and taste them, they would learn what the source of human nourishment is. If they would investigate further they would see that you can live quite well on traditional domestic crops such as rice, barley, rye, buckwheat, and vegetables, and they could decide simply that this is all Japanese agriculture needs to grow. If that is all the farmers have to grow, farming becomes very easy.

Until now the line of thought among modern economists has been that small scale, self-sufficient farming is wrong—that this is a primitive kind of agriculture—one that should be eliminated as quickly as possible. It is being said that the area of each field must be expanded to handle the changeover to large-scale, American-style agriculture. This way of thinking does not apply only to agriculture—developments in all areas are moving in this direction.

The goal is to have only a few people in farming. The agricultural authorities say that fewer people, using large, modern machinery can get greater yields from the same acreage. This is considered agricultural progress. After the War, between 70% and 80% of the

---

*Chinese bell flower, arrowroot *(kudzu)*, thoroughwort (a boneset), *valerianacea*, bush clover, wild fringed pink, and Japanese pampas grass.

people in Japan were farmers. This quickly changed to 50%, then 30%, 20%, and now the figure stands at around 14%. It is the intention of the Ministry of Agriculture to achieve the same level as in Europe and America, keeping less than 10% of the people as farmers and discouraging the rest.

In my opinion, if 100% of the people were farming it would be ideal. There is just a quarter-acre of arable land for each person in Japan. If each single person were given one quarter-acre, that is 1¼ acres to a family of five, that would be more than enough land to support the family for the whole year. If natural farming were practiced, a farmer would also have plenty of time for leisure and social activities within the village community. I think this is the most direct path toward making this country a happy, pleasant land.

## Simply Serve Nature and All Is Well

Extravagance of desire is the fundamental cause which has led the world into its present predicament.

Fast rather than slow, more rather than less—this flashy "development" is linked directly to society's impending collapse. It has only served to separate man from nature. Humanity must stop indulging the desire for material possessions and personal gain and move instead toward spiritual awareness.

Agriculture must change from large mechanical operations to small farms attached only to life itself. Material life and diet should be given a simple place. If this is done, work becomes pleasant, and spiritual breathing space becomes plentiful.

The more the farmer increases the scale of his operation, the more his body and spirit are dissipated and the further he falls away from a spiritually satisfying life. A life of small-scale farming may appear to be primitive, but in living such a life, it becomes possible to contemplate the Great Way.* I believe that if one fathoms deeply one's own neighborhood and the everyday world in which he lives, the greatest of worlds will be revealed.

At the end of the year the one-acre farmer of long ago spent January, February, and March hunting rab-

---

*The path of spiritual awareness which involves attentiveness to and care for the ordinary activities of daily life.

bits in the hills. Though he was called a poor peasant, he still had this kind of freedom. The New Year's holiday lasted about three months. Gradually this vacation came to be shortened to two months, one month, and now New Year's has come to be a three-day holiday.

The dwindling of the New Year's holiday indicates how busy the farmer has become and how he has lost his easy-going physical and spiritual well-being. There is no time in modern agriculture for a farmer to write a poem or compose a song.

The other day I was surprised to notice, while I was cleaning the little village shrine, that there were some plaques hanging on the wall. Brushing off the dust and looking at the dim and faded letters, I could make out dozens of *haiku* poems. Even in a little village such as this, twenty or thirty people had composed *haiku* and presented them as offerings. That is how much open space people had in their lives in the old days. Some of the verses must have been several centuries old. Since it was that long ago they were probably poor farmers, but they still had leisure to write *haiku*.

Now there is no one in this village with enough time to write poetry. During the cold winter months, only a few villagers can find the time to sneak out for a day or two to go after rabbits. For leisure, now, the television is the center of attention, and there is no time at all for the simple pastimes which brought richness to the farmer's daily life. This is what I mean when I say that agriculture has become poor and weak spiritually; it is concerning itself only with material development.

Lao Tzu, the Taoist sage, says that a whole and decent life can be lived in a small village. Bodhidharma, the founder of Zen, spent nine years living in a cave without bustling about. To be worried about making money, expanding, developing, growing cash crops and shipping them out is not the way of the farmer. To be here, caring for a small field, in full possession of the freedom and plentitude of each day, every day—this must have been the original way of agriculture.

To break experience in half and call one side physical and the other spiritual is narrowing and confusing. People do not live dependent on food. Ultimately, we cannot know what food is. It would be better if people stopped even thinking about food. Similarly, it would be well if people stopped troubling themselves about discovering the "true meaning of life;" we can never know the answers to great spiritual questions, but *it's all right not to understand.* We have been born and are living on the earth to face directly the reality of living.

Living is no more than the result of being born. Whatever it is people eat to live, whatever people think they must eat to live, is nothing more than

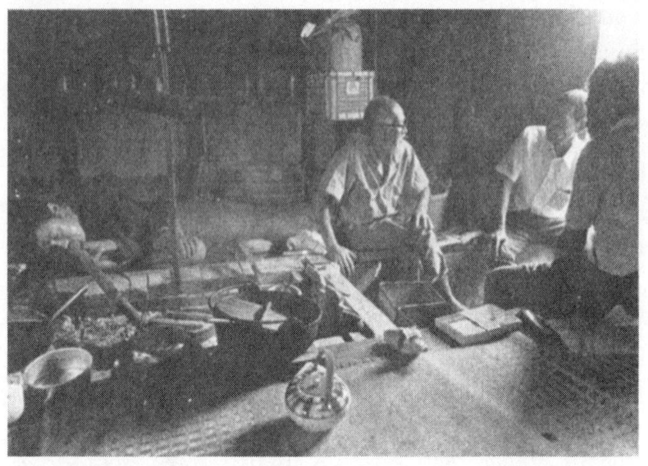

"There is no time in modern agriculture for a farmer to write a poem or compose a song."

something they have thought up. The world exists in such a way that if people will set aside their human will and be guided instead by nature there is no reason to expect to starve.

Just to live here and now—this is the true basis of human life. When a naive scientific knowledge becomes the basis of living, people come to live as if they are dependent only on starch, fats, and protein, and plants on nitrogen, phosphorous, and potash.

And the scientists, no matter how much they investigate nature, no matter how far they research, they only come to realize in the end how perfect and mysterious nature really is. To believe that by research and invention humanity can create something better than nature is an illusion. I think that people are struggling for no other reason than to come to know what you might call the vast incomprehensibility of nature.

So for the farmer in his work: serve nature and all is well. Farming used to be sacred work. When humanity fell away from this ideal, modern commercial agriculture rose. When the farmer began to grow crops to make money, he forgot the real principles of agriculture.

Of course the merchant has a role to play in society, but glorification of merchant activities tends to draw people away from a recognition of the true source of life. Farming, as an occupation which is within nature, lies close to this source. Many farmers are unaware of nature even while living and working in natural surroundings, but it seems to me that farming offers many opportunities for greater awareness.

"Whether autumn will bring wind or rain, I cannot know, but today I will be working in the fields." Those are the words of an old country song. They express the truth of farming as a way of life. No matter how the harvest will turn out, whether or not there will be enough food to eat, in simply sowing seed and caring tenderly for plants under nature's guidance there is joy.

## Various Schools of Natural Farming

I do not particularly like the word "work." Human beings are the only animals who have to work, and I think this is the most ridiculous thing in the world. Other animals make their livings by living, but people work like crazy, thinking that they have to in order to stay alive. The bigger the job, the greater the challenge, the more wonderful they think it is. It would be good to give up that way of thinking and live an easy, comfortable life with plenty of free time. I think that the way animals live in the tropics, stepping outside in the morning and evening to see if there is something to eat, and taking a long nap in the afternoon, must be a wonderful life.

For human beings, a life of such simplicity would be possible if one worked to produce directly his daily necessities. In such a life, work is not work as people generally think of it, but simply doing what needs to be done.

To move things in this direction is my goal. It is also the goal of the seven or eight young people who live communally in the huts on the mountain and help out with the farming chores. These young people want to become farmers, to establish new villages and communities, and to give this sort of life a try. They come to my farm to learn the practical skills of farming that they will need to carry out this plan.

If you look across the country you might notice that quite a few communes have been springing up recently. If they are called gatherings of hippies, well, they could be viewed that way too, I suppose. But in living and working together, finding the way back to nature, they are the model of the "new farmer." They understand that to become firmly rooted means to live from the yields of their own land. A community that cannot manage to produce its own food will not last long.

Many of these young people travel to India, or to France's Gandhi Village, spend time on a *kibbutz* in Israel, or visit communes in the mountains and deserts of the American West. There are those like the group on Suwanose Island in the Tokara Island chain of Southern Japan, who try new forms of family living and experience the closeness of tribal ways. I think that the movement of this handful of people is leading the way to a better time. It is among these people that natural farming is now rapidly taking hold and gaining momentum.

In addition, various religious groups have come to take up natural farming. In seeking the essential nature of man, no matter how you go about it, you must begin with the consideration of health. The path which leads to right awareness involves living each day straightforwardly and growing and eating wholesome, natural food. It follows that natural farming has been for many people the best place to begin.

I do not belong to any religious group myself and will freely discuss my views with anyone at all. I do not care much for making distinctions among Christianity, Buddhism, Shinto, and the other religions, but it does intrigue me that people of deep religious conviction are attracted to my farm. I think this is because natural farming, unlike other types of farming, is based on a philosophy which penetrates beyond considerations of soil analysis, pH, and harvest yields.

Some time ago, a fellow from the Paris Organic Gardening Center climbed up the mountain, and we spent the day talking. Hearing about affairs in France, I learned that they were planning an organic farming conference on an international scale, and as preparation for the meeting, this Frenchman was visiting organic and natural farms all over the world. I showed him around the orchard and then we sat down over a cup of mugwort tea and discussed some of my observations over the past thirty-odd years.

First I said that when you look over the principles of the organic farming popular in the West, you will find that they hardly differ from those of the traditional Oriental agriculture practiced in China, Korea, and Japan for many centuries. All Japanese farmers were still using this type of farming through the Meiji and Taisho Eras* and right up until the end of the Second World War.

It was a system which emphasized the fundamental importance of compost and of recycling human and animal waste. The form of management was intensive and included such practices as crop rotation, companion planting, and the use of green manure. Since space was limited, fields were never left untended and the planting and harvesting schedules proceeded with precision. All organic residue was made into compost and returned to the fields. The use of compost was officially encouraged and agricultural research was mainly concerned with organic matter and composting techniques.

So an agriculture joining animals, crops, and human beings into one body existed as the mainstream of Japanese farming up to modern times. It could be said that organic farming as practiced in the

---

*1868-1926.

West takes as its point of departure this traditional agriculture of the Orient.

I went on to say that among natural farming methods two kinds could be distinguished: broad, transcendent natural farming, and the narrow natural farming of the relative world.* If I were pressed to talk about it in Buddhist terms, the two could be called respectively as Mahayana and Hinayana natural farming.

Broad, Mahayana natural farming arises of itself when a unity exists between man and nature. It conforms to nature as it is, and to the mind as it is. It proceeds from the conviction that if the individual temporarily abandons human will and so allows himself to be guided by nature, nature responds by providing everything. To give a simple analogy, in transcendent natural farming the relationship between humanity and nature can be compared with a husband and wife joined in perfect marriage. The marriage is not bestowed, not received; the perfect pair comes into existence of itself.

Narrow natural farming, on the other hand, is *pursuing* the way of nature; it self-consciously *attempts*, by "organic" or other methods, to follow nature. Farming is used for achieving a given objective. Although sincerely loving nature and earnestly proposing to her, the relationship is still tentative. Modern industrial farming desires heaven's wisdom, without grasping its meaning, and at the same time wants to make use of nature. Restlessly searching, it is unable to find anyone to propose to.

The narrow view of natural farming says that it is good for the farmer to apply organic material to the soil and good to raise animals, and that this is the best and most efficient way to put nature to use. To speak

*This is the world as understood by the intellect.

in terms of personal practice, this is fine, but with this way alone, the spirit of true natural farming cannot be kept alive. This kind of narrow natural farming is analogous to the school of swordsmanship known as the one-stroke school, which seeks victory through the skillful, yet self-conscious application of technique. Modern industrial farming follows the two-stroke school, which believes that victory can be won by delivering the greatest barrage of swordstrokes.

Pure natural farming, by contrast, is the no-stroke school. It goes nowhere and seeks no victory. Putting "doing nothing" into practice is the one thing the farmer should strive to accomplish. Lao Tzu spoke of non-active nature, and I think that if he were a farmer he would certainly practice natural farming. I believe that Gandhi's way, a methodless method, acting with a non-winning, non-opposing state of mind, is akin to natural farming. When it is understood that one loses joy and happiness in the attempt to possess them, the essence of natural farming will be realized. The ultimate goal of farming is not the growing of crops, but the cultivation and perfection of human beings.*

---

*In this paragraph Mr. Fukuoka is drawing a distinction between techniques undertaken in conscious pursuit of a given objective, and those which arise spontaneously as the expression of a person's harmony with nature as he goes about his daily business, free from the domination of the volitional intellect.

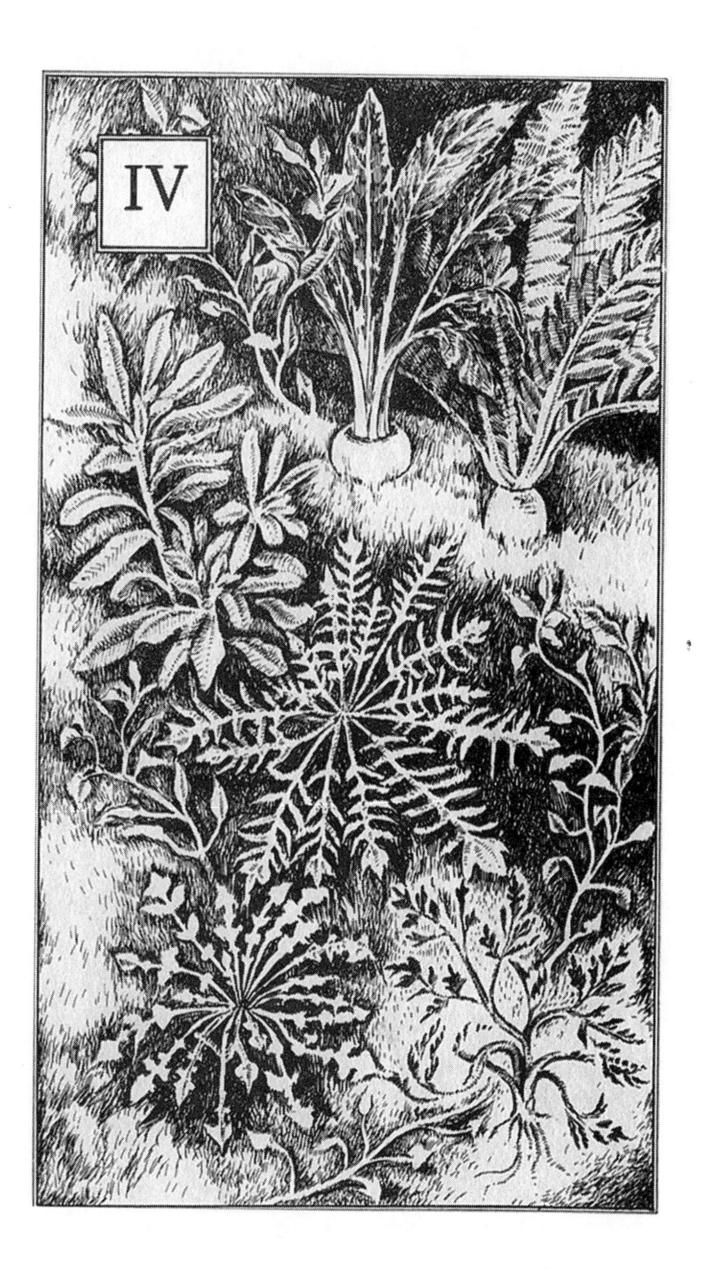
IV

## Confusion about Food

A young fellow who had stayed three years in one of the huts on the mountain said one day, "You know, when people say 'natural food' I don't know what they mean any more."

When you think about it, everybody is familiar with the words "natural food," but it is not clearly understood what natural food actually is. There are many who feel that eating food which contains no artificial chemicals or additives is a natural diet, and there are others who think vaguely that a natural diet is eating foods just as they are found in nature.

If you ask whether the use of fire and salt in cooking is natural or unnatural, one could answer either way. If the diet of the people of primitive times, eating only plants and animals living in their wild state, is "natural," then a diet which uses salt and fire cannot be called natural. But if it is argued that the knowledge acquired in ancient times of using fire and salt was humanity's natural destiny, then food prepared accordingly is perfectly natural. Is food to which human techniques of preparation have been applied good, or should wild foods just as they are in nature be considered good? Can cultivated crops be said to be natural? Where do you draw the line between natural and unnatural?

It could be said that the term "natural diet" in

Japan originated with the teachings of Sagen Ishizuka in the Meiji Era. His theory was later refined and elaborated by Mr. Sakurazawa* and Mr. Niki. The Path of Nutrition, known in the West as Macrobiotics, is based on the theory of non-duality and the yin-yang concepts of the I Ching. Since this usually means a brown rice diet, "natural diet" is generally thought of as eating whole grains and vegetables. Natural food, however, cannot be summed up so simply as brown rice vegetarianism.

So what is it?

The reason for all the confusion is that there are two paths of human knowledge—discriminating and non-discriminating.** People generally believe that unmistaken recognition of the world is possible through discrimination alone. Therefore, the word "nature" as it is generally spoken, denotes nature as it is perceived by the discriminating intellect.

I deny the empty image of nature as created by the human intellect, and clearly distinguish it from nature itself as experienced by non-discriminating understanding. If we eradicate the false conception of nature, I believe the root of the world's disorder will disappear.

---

*George Osawa.

**This is a distinction made by many Oriental philosophers. Discriminating knowledge is derived from the analytic, willful intellect in an attempt to organize experience into a logical framework. Mr. Fukuoka believes that in this process, the individual sets himself apart from nature. It is the "limited scientific truth and judgment" discussed on pg. 84.

Non-discriminating knowledge arises without conscious effort on the part of the individual when experience is accepted as it is, without interpretation by the intellect.

While discriminating knowledge is essential for analyzing practical problems in the world, Mr. Fukuoka believes that ultimately it provides too narrow a perspective.

In the West natural science developed from discriminating knowledge; in the East the philosophy of yin-yang and of the I Ching developed from the same source. But scientific truth can never reach absolute truth, and philosophies, after all, are nothing more than interpretations of the world. Nature as grasped by scientific knowledge is a nature which has been destroyed; it is a ghost possessing a skeleton, but no soul. Nature as grasped by philosophical knowledge is a theory created out of human speculation, a ghost with a soul, but no structure.

There is no way in which non-discriminating knowledge can be realized except by direct intuition, but people try to fit it into a familiar framework by calling it "instinct". It is actually knowledge from an unnamable source. Abandon the discriminating mind and transcend the world of relativity if you want to know the true appearance of nature. From the beginning there is no east or west, no four seasons, and no yin or yang.

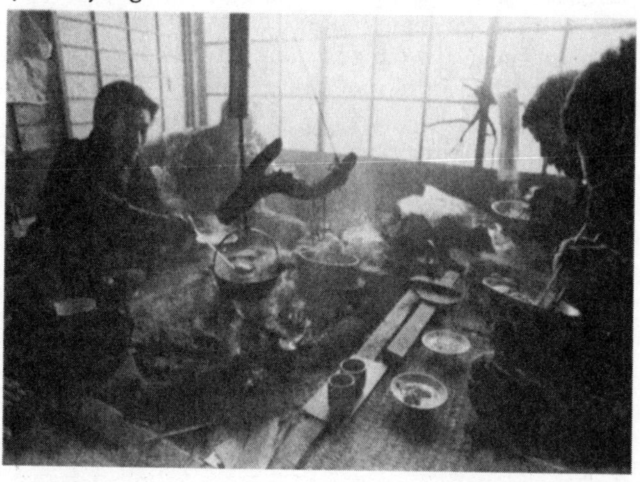

A mid-day meal of soup and rice with pickled vegetables.

When I had gone this far, the youth asked, "Then you not only deny natural science, but also the Oriental philosophies based on yin-yang and the I Ching?"

As temporary expedients or as directional markers they could be acknowledged as valuable, I said, but they should not be considered as the highest achievements. Scientific truths and philosophies are concepts of the relative world, and there they hold true and their value is recognized. For example, for modern people living in the relative world, disrupting the order of nature and bringing about the collapse of their own body and spirit, the yin-yang system can serve as a fitting and effective pointer toward the restoration of order.

Such paths could be said to be useful theories to help people achieve a condensed and compact diet until a true natural diet is attained. But if you realize that the eventual human goal is to transcend the world of relativity, to play in a realm of freedom, then plodding along attached to theory is unfortunate. When the individual is able to enter a world in which the two aspects of yin and yang return to their original unity, the mission of these symbols comes to an end.

A youth who had recently arrived spoke up: "Then if you become a natural person you can eat anything you want?"

If you expect a bright world on the other side of the tunnel, the darkness of the tunnel lasts all the longer. When you no longer *want* to eat something tasty, you can taste the real flavor of whatever you are eating. It is easy to lay out the simple foods of a natural diet on the dining table, but those who can truly enjoy such a feast are few.

# Nature's Food Mandala

My thinking on natural food is the same as it is on natural farming. Just as natural farming complies with nature as it is, that is, nature as apprehended by the non-discriminating mind, so natural diet is a way of eating in which foods gathered in the wild or crops grown through natural farming, and fish caught by natural methods, are acquired without intentional action through the non-discriminating mind.

Even though I speak of non-intentional action and non-method, wisdom acquired over time in the course of daily life is, of course, acknowledged. The use of salt and fire in cooking could be criticized as the first step in the separation of man from nature, but it is simply natural wisdom as apprehended by primitive people, and should be sanctioned as wisdom bestowed by heaven.

Crops which have evolved over thousands and tens of thousands of years by dwelling together with human beings are not products born entirely from the discriminating knowledge of the farmer, and can be thought of as naturally occurring foods. But the instantly altered varieties which have not evolved under natural circumstances, but rather have been developed by an agricultural science which has drawn far away from nature, as well as mass-produced fish, shellfish, and domestic animals, fall outside that category.

Farming, fishing, animal raising, the everyday realities of food, clothing, shelter, spiritual life—everything there is—must form a union with nature.

I have drawn the following diagrams to help explain the natural diet which transcends science and philosophy. The first brings together the foods which people can most easily obtain, and these are arranged more or less in groups. The second shows the foods as they are available during the various months of the year. These diagrams compose nature's food mandala.* From this mandala it can be seen that the sources of food provided on the face of the earth are nearly limitless. If people will acquire food through "no-mind",** even though they know nothing at all about yin and yang, they can attain a perfect natural diet.

The fishermen and farmers in a Japanese village have no particular interest in the logic of these diagrams. They follow nature's prescription by selecting seasonal foods from their immediate area.

From early spring, when the seven herbs sprout forth from the earth, the farmer can taste seven flavors. To go along with these are the delicious flavors of pond snails, sea clams, and turban shellfish.

The season of green arrives in March. Horsetail, bracken, mugwort, osmund, and other mountain plants, and of course the young leaves of the persimmon and peach trees and the sprouts of mountain yams can all be eaten. Possessing a light, delicate flavor, they make delicious tempura and can also be used as seasonings. At the seashore, sea vegetables such as kelp, *nori,* and rockweed are delicious and abundant during the spring months.

---

*A circular diagram in eastern art and religion, symbolizing the totality and wholeness of its subject.

**A Buddhist term which describes the state in which there is no distinction between the individual and the "external" world.

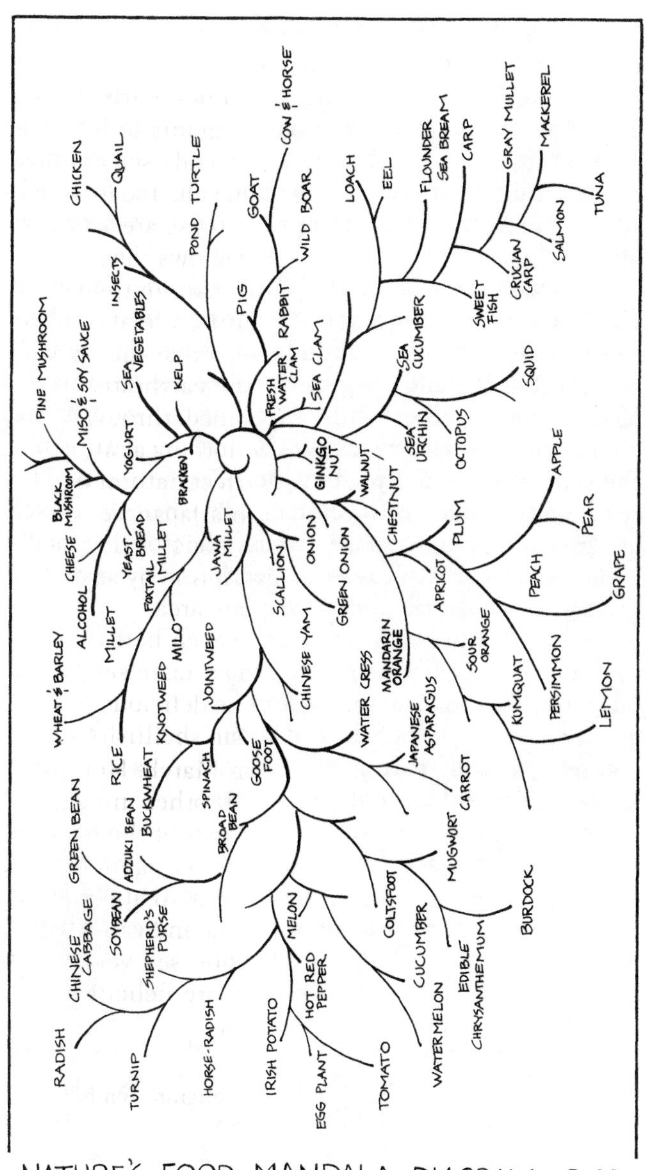


NATURE'S FOOD MANDALA DIAGRAM ONE

When the bamboo sends up its young shoots, grey rock cod, sea bream, and striped pig fish are at their most delicious. The iris blossom season is celebrated with the slender ribbon fish and mackerel *sashimi*. Green peas, snow peas, lima beans, and fava beans are delicious eaten right from the pod or boiled with whole grains such as brown rice, wheat, or barley.

Toward the end of the rainy season,* Japanese plums are salted away, and strawberries and raspberries can be gathered in abundance. At this time it is natural that the body begins to desire the crisp flavor of scallions together with watery fruits such as loquats, apricots, and peaches. The loquat's fruit is not the only part of the plant which can be eaten. The seed can be ground into "coffee," and when the leaves are brewed to make tea it is among the finest of medicines. The mature leaves of peach and persimmon trees produce a tonic for longevity.

Beneath the bright midsummer sun, eating melons and licking honey in the shade of a big tree is a favorite pastime. The many summer vegetables such as carrot, spinach, radish, and cucumber become ripe and ready for harvesting. The body also needs vegetable or sesame oil to hold off summer sloth.

If you call it mysterious, then mysterious it is that the winter grain harvested in spring goes well with the decreased summertime appetite, and so in summer barley noodles of various sizes and shapes are prepared often. Buckwheat grain is harvested in summer. It is an ancient wild plant and a food which goes well with this season.

Early fall is a happy season, with soybeans and small red *azuki* beans, many fruits, vegetables, and various yellow grains all ripening at the same time.

---

*In most of Japan the rainy season lasts from June to mid-July.

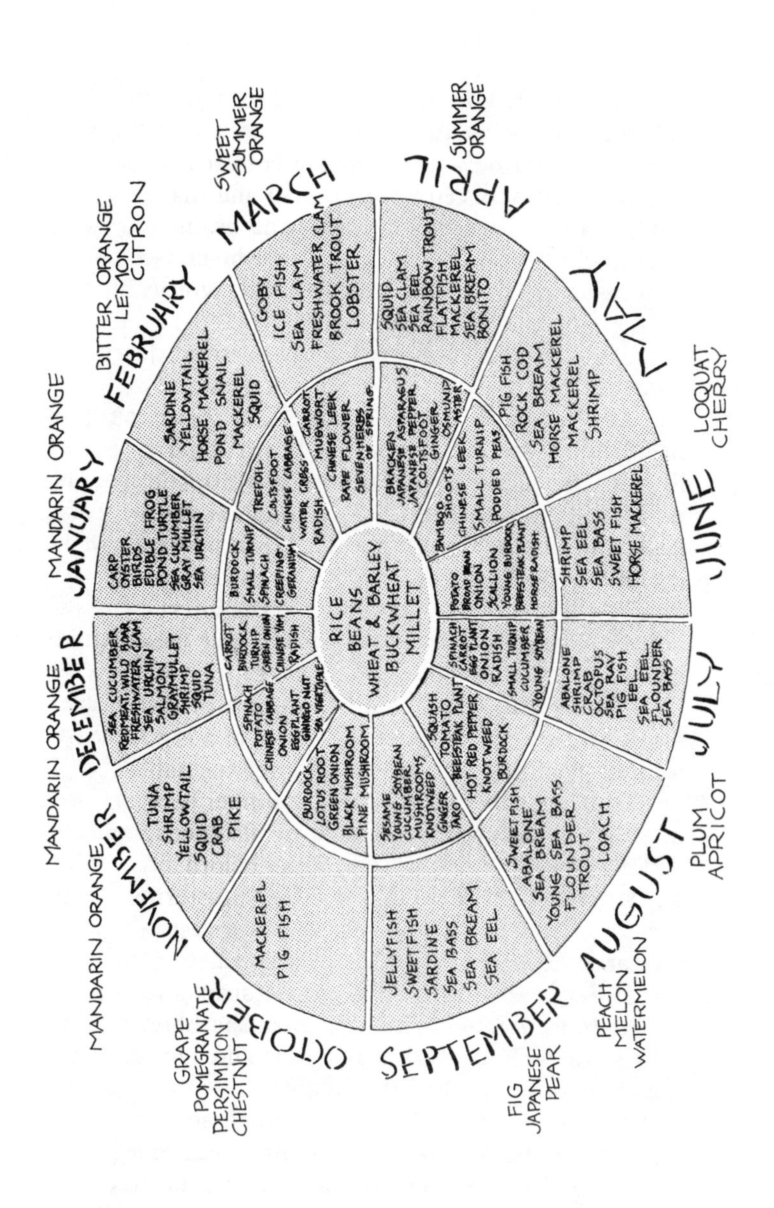


NATURE'S FOOD MANDALA DIAGRAM TWO

Millet cakes are enjoyed at the autumn moon viewing celebrations. Parboiled soybeans are served along with taro potatoes. As autumn deepens, maize, and rice steamed with red beans, *matsutake* mushrooms, or chestnuts are eaten and enjoyed often. Most important, the rice which has absorbed the sun's rays all summer long ripens in the fall. This means that a staple food which can be plentifully obtained and is rich in calories is provided for the cold winter months.

At first frost one feels like looking in on the fish-broiler's stand. Deep-water blue fish such as yellowtail and tuna can be caught during this season. It is interesting that the Japanese radish and the leafy vegetables abundant during this season go well with these fish.

The New Year's holiday cooking is prepared largely from food which has been pickled and salted away especially for the great celebration. Salted salmon, herring eggs, red sea bream, lobster, kelp, and black beans have been served every year at this feast for many centuries.

Digging the radishes and turnips which have been left in the ground, covered with a blanket of soil and snow, is an enjoyable experience during the winter season. Grains and various beans grown during the year and *miso* and soy sauce are staples always on hand. Along with the cabbages, radishes, squash, and sweet potatoes stored in the autumn, a variety of foods are available during the months of bitter cold. Leeks and wild scallions go well with the delicate flavor of oysters and sea cucumbers which can be gathered then.

Waiting for spring to arrive, one catches sight of colt's foot shoots and the edible leaves of the creeping strawberry geranium peeping out of the snow. With the return of watercress, shepherd's purse, chickweed, and the other wild herbs, a garden of natural spring vegetables can be harvested beneath the kitchen window.

Thus, by following a humble diet, gathering the foods of the various seasons from close at hand, and savoring their wholesome and nourishing flavor, the local villagers accept what nature provides.

The villagers know the delicious flavor of the food, but they cannot taste the mysterious flavor of nature. No, it is rather that they taste it, but cannot express it with words.

A natural diet lies right at one's feet.

# The Culture of Food

When asked why we eat food, few think further than the fact that food is necessary to support the life and growth of the human body. Beyond this, however, there is the deeper question of the relationship of food to the human spirit. For animals it is enough to eat, play, and sleep. For humans, too, it would be a great accomplishment if they could enjoy nourishing food, a simple daily round, and restful sleep.

Buddha said, "Form is emptiness and emptiness is form." Since the "form" of Buddhist terminology indicates matter, or things, and emptiness is the mind, he is saying that matter and mind are the same. Things have many different colors, shapes, and flavors, and people's minds flit from side to side, attracted to the various qualities of things. But actually, matter and mind are one.

## Color

In the world there are seven basic colors. But if these seven colors are combined, they become white. When split by a prism the white light becomes seven colors. When man views the world with "no-mind" the color in the color vanishes. It is no-color. Only when they are viewed by the seven-colored mind of discrimination do the seven colors appear.

Water undergoes countless changes but water is still water. In the same way, although the conscious mind appears to undergo changes, the original unmoving mind does not change. When one becomes infatuated with the seven colors, the mind is easily distracted. The colors of leaves, branches, and fruit are perceived, while the basis of color passes unnoticed.

This is also true of food. In this world there are many natural substances that are suitable for human food. These foods are distinguished by the mind and are thought to have good and bad qualities. People then consciously select what they think they must have. This process of selection impedes the recognition of the basis of human nourishment, which is what heaven prescribes for the place and season.

Nature's colors, like hydrangea blossoms, change easily. The body of nature is perpetual transformation. For the same reason that it is called infinite motion, it may also be considered non-moving motion. When reason is applied to selecting foods, one's understanding of nature becomes fixed and nature's transformations, such as the seasonal changes, are ignored.

The purpose of a natural diet is not to create knowledgeable people who can give sound explanations and skillfully select among the various foods, but to create unknowing people who take food without consciously making distinctions. This does not go against the way of nature. By realizing "no-mind," without becoming lost in the subtleties of form, accepting the color of the colorless as color, right diet begins.

## Flavor

People say, "You don't know what food tastes like until you try it." But even when you do try it, the food's flavor may vary, depending on time and circumstance and the dispositon of the person who is tasting.

If you ask a scientist what the substance of flavor is, he will try to define it by isolating the various components and by determining the proportions of sweet, sour, bitter, salty, and pungent. But flavor cannot be defined by analysis or even by the tip of the tongue. Even though the five flavors are perceived by the tongue, the impressions are collected and interpreted by the mind.

A natural person can achieve right diet because his instinct is in proper working order. He is satisfied with simple food; it is nutritious, tastes good, and is useful daily medicine. Food and the human spirit are united.

Modern people have lost their clear instinct and consequently have become unable to gather and enjoy the seven herbs of spring. They go out seeking a variety of flavors. Their diet becomes disordered, the gap between likes and dislikes widens, and their instinct becomes more and more bewildered. At this point people begin to apply strong seasonings to their food and to use elaborate cooking techniques, further deepening the confusion. Food and the human spirit have become estranged.

Most people today have even become separated from the flavor of rice. The whole grain is refined and processed, leaving only the tasteless starch. Polished rice lacks the unique fragrance and flavor of whole rice. Consequently, it requires seasonings and must be supplemented with side dishes or covered with sauce. People think, mistakenly, that it does not matter that the food value of the rice is low, as long as vitamin supplements or other foods such as meat or fish supply the missing nutrients.

Flavorful foods are not flavorful in themselves.

Food is not delicious unless a person thinks it is. Although most people think that beef and chicken are delectable, to a person who for physical or spiritual reasons has decided that he dislikes them, they are repulsive.

Just playing or doing nothing at all, children are happy. A discriminating adult, on the other hand, decides what will make him happy, and when these conditions are met he feels satisfied. Foods taste good to him not necessarily because they have nature's subtle flavors and are nourishing to the body, but because his taste has been conditioned to the *idea* that they taste good.

Wheat noodles are delicious, but a cup of instant noodles from a vending machine tastes extremely bad. But, by advertising, remove the idea that they taste bad, and to many people even these unsavory noodles somehow come to taste good.

There are stories that, deceived by a fox, people have eaten horse manure. It is nothing to laugh about. People nowadays eat with their minds, not with their bodies. Many people do not care if there is monosodium glutamate in their food, but they taste only with the tip of the tongue, so they are easily fooled.

At first people ate simply because they were alive and because food was tasty. Modern people have come to think that if they do not prepare food with elaborate seasonings, the meal will be tasteless. If you do not *try* to make food delicious, you will find that nature has made it so.

The first consideration should be to live in such a way that the food itself tastes good, but today all the effort goes instead into *adding* tastiness to food. Ironically, delicious foods have all but vanished.

People tried to make delicious bread, and delicious bread disappeared. In trying to make rich luxurious foods they made useless foods, and now people's appetites are unsatisfied.

The best methods of food preparation preserve nature's delicate flavors. The daily wisdom of long ago enabled people to make the various kinds of vegetable pickles, such as sun-dried pickles, salt-pickles, bran-pickles, and *miso*-pickles, so that the flavor of the vegetable itself was also preserved.

The art of cooking begins with sea salt and a crackling fire. When food is prepared by someone sensitive to the fundamentals of cookery, it maintains its natural flavor. If, by being cooked, food takes on some strange and exotic flavor, and if the purpose of this change is merely to delight the palate, this is false cooking.

Culture is usually thought of as something created, maintained, and developed by humanity's efforts alone. But culture always originates in the partnership of man and nature. When the union of human society and nature is realized, culture takes shape of itself. Culture has always been closely connected with daily life, and so has been passed on to future generations, and has been preserved up to the present time.

Something born from human pride and the quest for pleasure cannot be considered true culture. True culture is born within nature, and is simple, humble, and pure. Lacking true culture, humanity will perish.

When people rejected natural food and took up refined food instead, society set out on a path toward its own destruction. This is because such food is not the product of true culture. Food is life, and life must not step away from nature.

# Living by Bread Alone

There is nothing better than eating delicious food, but for most people eating is just a way to nourish the body, to have energy to work and to live to an old age. Mothers often tell their children to eat their food—even if they do not like the taste—because it is "good" for them.

But nutrition cannot be separated from the sense of taste. Nutritious foods, good for the human body, whet the appetite and are delicious on their own account. Proper nourishment is inseparable from good flavor.

Not too long ago the daily meal of the farmers in this area consisted of rice and barley with *miso* and pickled vegetables. This diet gave long life, a strong constitution, and good health. Stewed vegetables and steamed rice with red beans was a once-a-month feast. The farmer's healthy, robust body was able to nourish itself well on this simple rice diet.

The traditional brown rice-and-vegetable diet of the East is very different from that of most Western societies. Western nutritional science believes that unless certain amounts of starch, fat, protein, minerals, and vitamins are eaten each day, a well-balanced diet and good health cannot be preserved. This belief produced the mother who stuffs "nutritious" food into her youngster's mouth.

One might suppose that Western dietetics, with its elaborate theories and calculations, could leave no doubts about proper diet. The fact is, it creates far more problems than it resolves.

One problem is that in Western nutritional science there is no effort to adjust the diet to the natural cycle. The diet that results serves to isolate human beings from nature. A fear of nature and a general sense of insecurity are often the unfortunate results.

Another problem is that spiritual and emotional values are entirely forgotten, even though foods are directly connected with human spirit and emotions. If the human being is viewed merely as a physiological object, it is impossible to produce a coherent understanding of diet. When bits and pieces of informa-

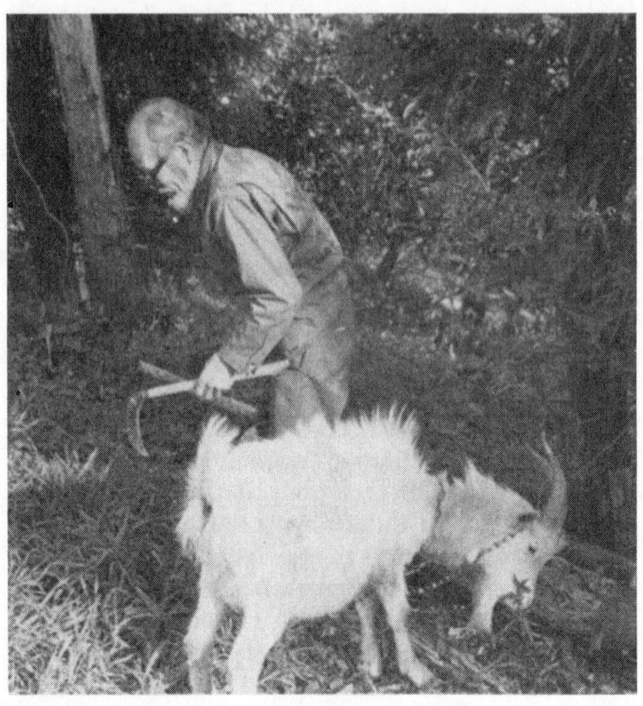

tion are collected and brought together in confusion, the result is an imperfect diet which draws away from nature.

"Within one thing lie all things, but if all things are brought together not one thing can arise." Western science is unable to grasp this precept of eastern philosophy. A person can analyze and investigate a butterfly as far as he likes, but he cannot make a butterfly.

If the Western scientific diet were put into practice on a wide scale, what sort of practical problems do you suppose would occur? High quality beef, eggs, milk, vegetables, bread, and other foods would have to be readily available all year around. Large scale production and long-term storage would become necessary. Already in Japan, adoption of this diet has caused farmers to produce summer vegetables such as lettuce, cucumbers, eggplants, and tomatoes in the winter. It will not be long before farmers are asked to harvest persimmons in spring and peaches in the autumn.

It is unreasonable to expect that a wholesome, balanced diet can be achieved simply by supplying a great variety of foods regardless of the season. Compared with plants which ripen naturally, vegetables and fruits grown out-of-season under necessarily unnatural conditions contain few vitamins and minerals. It is not surprising that summer vegetables grown in the autumn or winter have none of the flavor and fragrance of those grown beneath the sun by organic and natural methods.

Chemical analysis, nutritional ratios, and other such considerations are the main causes of error. The food prescribed by modern science is far from the traditional Oriental diet, and it is undermining the health of the Japanese people.

## Summing Up Diet

In this world there exist four main classifications of diet:

(1) A lax diet conforming to habitual desires and taste preferences. People following this diet sway back and forth erratically in response to whims and fancies. This diet could be called self-indulgent, empty eating.

(2) The standard nutritional diet of most people, proceeding from biological conclusions. Nutritious foods are eaten for the purpose of maintaining the life of the body. It could be called materialist, scientific eating.

(3) The diet based on spiritual principles and idealistic philosophy. Limiting foods, aiming toward compression, most "natural" diets fall into this category. This could be called the diet of principle.

(4) The natural diet, following the will of heaven. Discarding all human knowledge, this diet could be called the diet of non-discrimination.

People first draw away from the empty diet which is the source of countless diseases. Next, becoming disenchanted with the scientific diet, which merely attempts to maintain biological life, many proceed to a diet of principle. Finally, transcending this, one arrives at the non-discriminating diet of the natural person.

## The Diet of Non-Discrimination

Human life is not sustained by its own power. Nature gives birth to human beings and keeps them alive. This is the relation in which people stand to nature. Food is a gift of heaven. People do not create foods from nature; heaven bestows them.

Food is food and food is not food. It is a part of man and is apart from man.

When food, the body, the heart, and the mind become perfectly united within nature, a natural diet becomes possible. The body as it is, following its own instinct, eating if something tastes good, abstaining if it does not, is free.

It is impossible to prescribe rules and proportions for a natural diet.* This diet defines itself according to the local environment, and the various needs and the bodily constitution of each person.

## The Diet of Principle

Everyone should be aware that nature is always complete, balanced in perfect harmony within itself. Natural food is whole and within the whole are nourishment and subtle flavors.

It appears that, by applying the system of yin and yang, people can explain the origin of the universe and the transformations of nature. It may also seem that the harmony of the human body can be deter-

*A definite code or system by which one can consciously decide these questions is impossible. Nature, or the body itself, serves as a capable guide. But this subtle guidance goes unheard by most people because of the clamor caused by desire and by the activity of the discriminating mind.

mined and consciously sustained. But if the doctrines are entered into too deeply (as is necessary in the study of Eastern medicine) one enters the domain of science and fails to make the essential escape from discriminating perception.

Swept along by the subtleties of human knowledge without recognizing its limits, the practitioner of the diet of principle comes to concern himself only with separate objects. But when trying to grasp the meaning of nature with a wide and far-reaching vision, he fails to notice the small things happening at his feet.

## The Typical Sick Person's Diet

Sickness comes when people draw apart from nature. The severity of the disease is directly proportional to the degree of separation. If a sick person returns to a healthy environment often the disease will disappear. When alienation from nature becomes extreme, the number of sick people increases. Then the desire to return to nature becomes stronger. But in *seeking* to return to nature, there is no clear understanding of what nature is, and so the attempt proves futile.

Even if one lives a primitive life back in the mountains, he may still fail to grasp the true objective. If you *try* to do something, your efforts will never achieve the desired result.

People living in the cities face tremendous difficulty in trying to attain a natural diet. Natural food is simply not available, because farmers have stopped growing it. Even if they could buy natural food, people's bodies would need to be fit to digest such hearty fare.

In this sort of situation, if you try to eat wholesome meals or attain a balanced yin-yang diet, you need practically supernatural means and powers of judgment. Far from a return to nature, a complicated, strange sort of "natural" diet arises and the individual is only drawn further away from nature.

If you look inside "health food" stores these days you will find a bewildering assortment of fresh foods, packaged foods, vitamins, and dietary supplements. In the literature many different types of diets are presented as being "natural," nutritious, and the best for health. If someone says it is healthful to boil foods together, there is someone else who says foods boiled together are only good for making people sick. Some emphasize the essential value of salt in the diet, others say that too much salt causes disease. If there is someone who shuns fruit as yin and food for monkeys, there is someone else who says fruit and vegetables are the very best foods for providing longevity and a happy disposition.

At various times and in various circumstances all of these opinions could be said to be correct, and so people come to be confused. Or rather, to a confused person, all of these theories become material for creating greater confusion.

Nature is in constant transition, changing from moment to moment. People cannot grasp nature's true appearance. The face of nature is unknowable. Trying to capture the unknowable in theories and formalized doctrines is like trying to catch the wind in a butterfly net.

If you hit the mark on the wrong target, you have missed.

Humanity is like a blind man who does not know where he is heading. He gropes around with the cane of scientific knowledge, depending on yin and yang to set his course.

What I want to say is, don't eat food with your head, and that is to say get rid of the discriminating mind. I hoped that the food mandala I drew earlier would serve as a guide to show at a glance the relationship of various foods to each other and to human beings. But you can throw that away too after you have seen it once.

The prime consideration is for a person to develop the sensitivity to allow the body to choose food by itself. Thinking only about the foods themselves and leaving the spirit aside, is like making visits to the temple, reading the sutras, and leaving Buddha on the outside. Rather than studying philosophical theory to reach an understanding of food, it is better to arrive at a theory from *within* one's daily diet.

Doctors take care of sick people; healthy people are cared for by nature. Instead of getting sick and then becoming absorbed in a natural diet to get well, one should live in a natural environment so that sickness does not appear.

The young people who come to stay in the huts on the mountain and live a primitive life, eating natural foods and practicing natural farming, are aware of man's ultimate purpose, and they have set out to live in accordance with it in the most direct way.

# Food and Farming

This book on natural farming necessarily includes a consideration of natural food. This is because food and farming are the front and back of one body. It is clearer than firelight that if natural farming is not practiced natural food will not be available to the public. But if natural diet is not established the farmer will remain confused about what to grow.

Unless people become natural people, there can be neither natural farming nor natural food. In one of the huts on the mountain I left the words, "Right Food, Right Action, Right Awareness"* inscribed on a pinewood plaque above the fireplace. The three cannot be separated from one another. If one is missing, none can be realized. If one is realized, all are realized.

People complacently view the world as a place where "progress" grows out of turmoil and confusion. But purposeless and destructive development invites confusion of thought, invites nothing less than the degeneration and collapse of humankind. If it is not clearly understood what the non-moving source of all this activity is—what nature is—it will be impossible to recover our health.

---

*This motto is phrased after the Buddhist Eightfold Path of spiritual realization.

# V

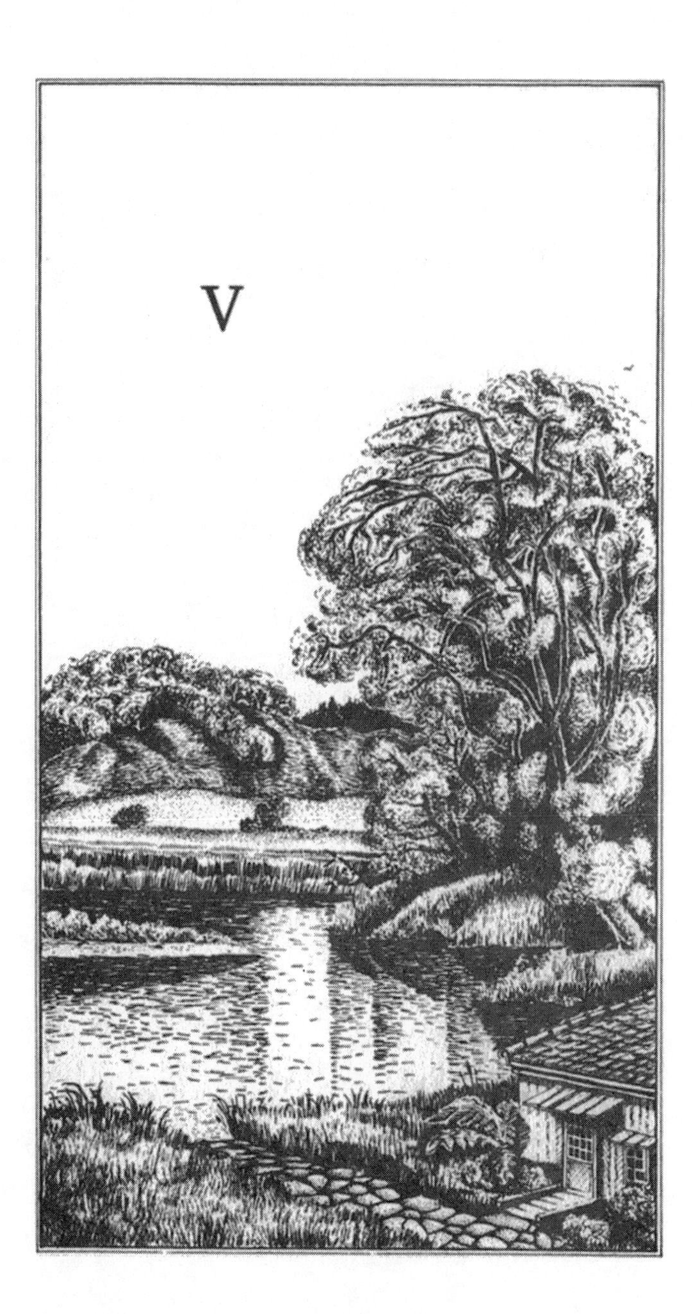

# Foolishness Comes Out Looking Smart

The autumn nights are long and chilly. The time would be well spent gazing into glowing coals, hands pressed around a warm cup of tea. It is said that anything is fine to talk about while sitting around the fire, and so, thinking that the grudges of my fellow farmers would be an interesting topic, I have casually brought up the subject. But it seems there are going to be some problems.

Here I have been, talking all the time about how everything is of no account, saying that humanity is ignorant, that there is nothing to strive for, and that whatever is done is wasted effort. How can I say that and then go on chattering like this? If I push myself to write something, the only thing to write is that writing is useless. It is very perplexing.

I do not care to dwell on my own past long enough to write about it, and I am not wise enough to predict the future. Stirring the fire while making hearthside conversation on daily affairs, how can I ask anybody to put up with an old farmer's foolish notions?

On the ridgetop of the orchard, overlooking Matsuyama Bay and the broad Dogo Plain, are several small, mudwalled huts. There, a handful of people have gathered and are living a simple life together.

There are no modern conveniences. Spending peaceful evenings beneath candle and lamplight, they live a life of simple necessities: brown rice, vegetables, a robe and a bowl. They come from somewhere, stay for a while, and then move on.

Among the guests are agricultural researchers, students, scholars, farmers, hippies, poets and wanderers, young and old, men and women of various types and nationalities. Most of those who stay for a long time are young people in need of a period of introspection.

My function is to act as caretaker of this wayside inn, serving tea to the travellers who come and go. And while they are helping out in the fields, I enjoy listening to how things are going in the world.

This sounds fine, but actually it is not such a soft and easy life. I advocate "do-nothing" farming, and so many people come, thinking they will find a utopia where one can live without ever having to get out of bed. These people are in for a big surprise. Hauling water from the spring in the early morning fog, split-

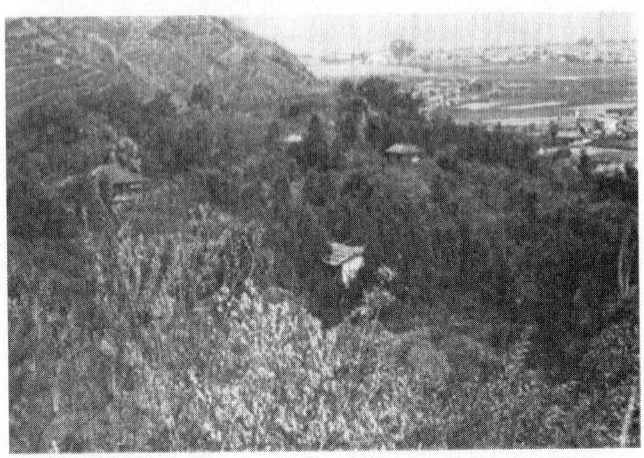

The orchard and huts from the mountain above.

ting firewood until their hands are red and stinging with blisters, working ankle-deep in mud—there are many who quickly call it quits.

Today, as I watched a group of young people work on a tiny hut, a young woman from Funabashi came walking up.

When I asked why she had come, she said, "I just came, that's all. I don't know anything anymore."

Bright young lady, nonchalant, has her wits about her.

I then asked, "If you know you are unenlightened, there is nothing to say, right? In coming to understand the world through the power of discrimination, people lose sight of its meaning. Isn't that why the world is in such a fix?"

She answered softly, "Yes, if you say so."

"Maybe you don't have a really clear idea of what enlightenment is. What kind of books did you read before coming here?"

She shook her head in rejection of reading.

People study because they think they do not understand, but studying is not going to help one to understand. They study hard only to find out in the end that people cannot know anything, that understanding lies beyond human reach.

Usually people think that the word "non-understanding" applies when you say, for example, that you understand nine things, but there is one thing you do not understand. But intending to understand ten things, you actually do not understand even one. If you know a hundred flowers you do not "know" a single one. People struggle hard to understand, convince themselves that they understand, and die knowing nothing.

The young people took a break from their carpentry, sat down on the grass near a big mandarin orange tree, and looked up at the wispy clouds in the southern sky.

People think that when they turn their eyes from the earth to the sky they see the heavens. They set the orange fruit apart from the green leaves and say they know the green of the leaves and the orange of the fruit. But from the instant one makes a distinction between green and orange, the true colors vanish.

People think they understand things because they become familiar with them. This is only superficial knowledge. It is the knowledge of the astronomer who knows the names of the stars, the botanist who knows the classification of the leaves and flowers, the artist who knows the aesthetics of green and red. This is not to know nature itself—the earth and sky, green and red. Astronomer, botanist, and artist have done no more than grasp impressions and interpret them, each within the vault of his own mind. The more involved they become with the activity of the intellect, the more they set themselves apart and the more difficult it becomes to live naturally.

The tragedy is that in their unfounded arrogance, people attempt to bend nature to their will. Human beings can destroy natural forms, but they cannot create them. Discrimination, a fragmented and incomplete understanding, always forms the starting point of human knowledge. Unable to know the whole of nature, people can do no better than to construct an incomplete model of it and then delude themselves into thinking that they have created something natural.

All someone has to do to know nature is to realize that he does not really *know* anything, that he is unable to know anything. It can then be expected that he will lose interest in discriminating knowledge. When he abandons discriminating knowledge, nondiscriminating knowledge of itself arises within him. If he does not try to think about knowing, if he does not care about understanding, the time will come when he will understand. There is no other way than through the destruction of the ego, casting aside the thought that humans exist apart from heaven and earth.

"This means being foolish instead of being smart," I snapped at a young fellow who had a wise look of complacency on his face. "What kind of look is that in your eyes? Foolishness comes out looking smart. Do you know for sure whether you're smart or foolish, or are you trying to become a foolish-type smart guy? You can't become smart, can't become foolish, stuck at a standstill. Isn't that where you are now?"

Before I knew it I was angry with myself for repeating the same words over and over again, words which could never match the wisdom of remaining silent, words I myself could not understand.

The autumn sun was sinking low on the horizon. Twilight colors approached the foot of the old tree. With the light from the Inland Sea at their backs, the silent youths returned slowly to the huts for their evening meal. I followed quietly behind in the shadows.

## Who Is the Fool?

It is said that there is no creature as wise as the human being. By applying this wisdom, people have become the only animals capable of nuclear war.

The other day the head of the natural foods store in front of Osaka Station climbed up the mountain, bringing along seven companions, like the seven gods of good fortune. At noon, while we were feasting on an impromptu brown rice hodgepodge, one of them told the following: "Among children there is always one without a care in the world who laughs happily as he pees, there is another who always ends up the 'horse' when playing 'horse and rider,' and always a third who is clever at tricking the others out of their afternoon snack. Before the head of the class is chosen, the teacher talks seriously about the desirable qualities of a good leader and the importance of making a wise decision. When the election is held, it is the youngster who laughs happily by the side of the road who is chosen."

Everyone was amused, but I could not understand why they were laughing. I thought it was only natural.

If things are seen in terms of gain and loss, one must regard as the loser the child who always ends up playing the role of the horse, but greatness and mediocrity do not apply to children. The teacher thought the clever child was the most remarkable, but the other children saw him as being clever in the wrong way, someone who would oppress others.

To think that the one who is smart and can look out for himself is exceptional, and that it is better to be exceptional, is to follow "adult" values. The one who goes about his own business, eats and sleeps well, the one with nothing to worry about, would seem to me to be living in the most satisfactory manner. There is no one so great as the one who does not try to accomplish anything.

In Aesop's fable, when the frogs asked god for a king, he presented them with a log. The frogs made fun of the dumb log and when they asked the god for a greater king, he sent down a crane. As the story goes, the crane pecked all the frogs to death.

If the one who stands out in front is great, the ones who follow behind have to struggle and strain. If you set a regular fellow up in front, those who come after have an easy time. People think that someone who is strong and clever is outstanding, and so they select a prime minister who pulls the country like a diesel locomotive.

"What kind of person should be chosen for prime minister?"

"A dumb log," I replied. "There's nobody better than *daruma-san,** " I replied. "He is such a relaxed fellow he can sit for years in meditation without saying a word. If you give him a shove he rolls over, but with the persistence of non-resistance he always sits back up. *Daruma-san* doesn't just sit idly by, keeping his hands and feet folded. Knowing that you *should* keep them folded, he scowls silently at the people who want to stick theirs out."

---

**Daruma-san* is a popular Japanese children's toy. It is a big balloon, weighted at the bottom, in the shape of a monk seated in meditation.

"If you did nothing at all the world could not keep running. What would the world be without development?"

"Why do you have to develop? If economic growth rises from 5% to 10%, is happiness going to double? What's wrong with a growth rate of 0%? Isn't this a rather stable kind of economics? Could there be anything better than living simply and taking it easy?"

People find something out, learn how it works, and put nature to use, thinking this will be for the good of humankind. The result of all this, up to now, is that the planet has become polluted, people have become confused, and we have invited in the chaos of modern times.

At this farm we practice "do-nothing" farming and eat wholesome and delicious grains, vegetables, and citrus. There is meaning and basic satisfaction

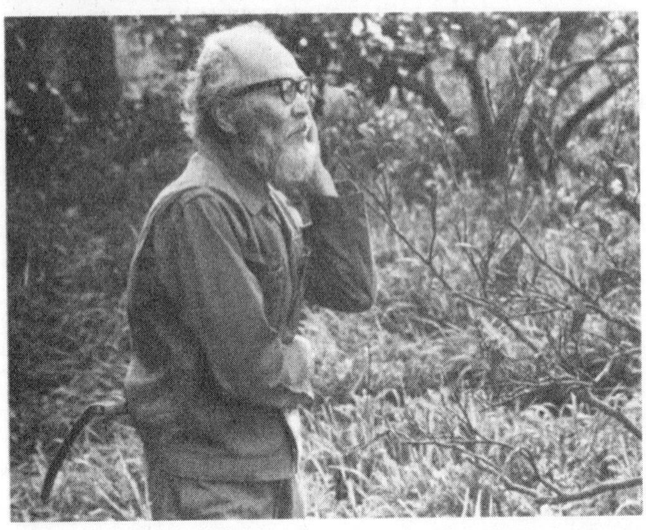

"We have come to the point at which there is no other way than to bring about a 'movement' not to bring anything about."

just in living close to the source of things. Life is song and poetry.

The farmer became too busy when people began to investigate the world and decided that it would be "good" if we did this or did that. All my research has been in the direction of *not* doing this or that. These thirty years have taught me that farmers would have been better off doing almost nothing at all.

The more people do, the more society develops, the more problems arise. The increasing desolation of nature, the exhaustion of resources, the uneasiness and disintegration of the human spirit, all have been brought about by humanity's trying to accomplish something. Originally there was no reason to progress, and nothing that had to be done. We have come to the point at which there is no other way than to bring about a "movement" not to bring anything about.

# I Was Born to Go to Nursery School

A young man with a small bag over his shoulder walked leisurely up to where we were working in the fields.

"Where are you from?" I asked.

"Over there."

"How did you get here?"

"I walked."

"What did you come here for?"

"I don't know."

Most of those who come here are in no hurry to reveal their names or the story of their past. They do not make their purpose very clear either. Since many of them do not know why they come, but just come, this is only natural.

From the first, man does not know where he comes from or where he is going. To say that you are born from your mother's womb and return to the earth is a biological explanation, but no one really knows what exists before birth or what kind of world is waiting after death.

Born without knowing the reason only to close one's eyes and depart for the infinite unknown—the human being is indeed a tragic creature.

The other day, I had found a woven sedge hat left by a group of pilgrims who were visiting the temples of Shikoku. On it were written the words, "Originally no east or west/ Ten infinite directions." Now, holding the hat in my hands, I asked the youth again where he had come from, and he said that he was the son of a temple priest in Kanazawa, and since it was just foolishness to read scriptures to the dead all day, he wanted to become a farmer.

There is no east or west. The sun comes up in the east, sets in the west, but this is merely an astronomical observation. Knowing that you do not understand either east or west is closer to the truth. The fact is, no one knows where the sun comes from.

Among the tens of thousands of scriptures, the one to be most grateful for, the one where all the important points are made, is the Heart Sutra. According to this sutra, "The Lord Buddha declared, 'Form is emptiness, emptiness is form. Matter and the spirit are one, but all is void. Man is not alive, is not dead, is unborn and undying, without old age and disease, without increase and without decrease.'"

The other day while we were cutting the rice, I said to the youths who were resting against a big pile of straw, "I was thinking that when rice is planted in the spring, the seed sends out living shoots, and now, as we are reaping, it appears to die. The fact that this ritual is repeated year after year means that life continues in this field and the yearly death is itself yearly birth. You could say that the rice we are cutting now lives continuously."

Human beings usually see life and death in a rather short perspective. What meaning can the birth of spring and the death of autumn have for this grass? People think that life is joy and death is sadness, but the rice seed, lying within the earth and sending out shoots in spring, its leaves and stems withering in the fall, still holds within its tiny core the full joy of life. The joy of life does not depart in death. Death is no more than a momentary passing. Wouldn't you say that this rice, because it possesses the full joyousness of life, does not know the sorrow of death?

The same thing that happens to rice and barley goes on continuously within the human body. Day by day hair and nails grow, tens of thousands of cells die, tens of thousands more are born; the blood in the body a month ago is not the same blood today. When you think that your own characteristics will be propagated in the bodies of your children and grandchil-children, you could say that you are dying and being reborn each day, and yet will live on for many generations after death.

If participation in this cycle can be experienced and savored each day, nothing more is necessary. But most people are not able to enjoy life as it passes and changes from day to day. They cling to life as they have already experienced it, and this habitual attachment brings fear of death. Paying attention only to the past, which has already gone, or to the future, which has yet to come, they forget that they are living on the earth here and now. Struggling in confusion, they watch their lives pass as in a dream.

"If life and death are realities, isn't human suffering inescapable?"

"There is no life or death."

"How can you say that?"

The world itself is a unity of matter within the flow of experience, but people's minds divide phenomena into dualities such as life and death, yin and yang, being and emptiness. The mind comes to believe in the absolute validity of what the senses perceive and then, for the first time, matter as it is turns into objects as human beings normally perceive them.

The forms of the material world, concepts of life and death, health and disease, joy and sorrow, all originate in the human mind. In the sutra, when Buddha said that all is void, he was not only denying intrinsic reality to anything which is constructed by human intellect, but he was also declaring that human emotions are illusions.

"You mean *all* is illusion? There's nothing left?"

"Nothing left? The concept of 'void' still remains in your mind apparently," I said to the youth. "If you don't know where you came from or where you're going, then how can you be sure you're here, standing in front of me? Is existence meaningless?"

". . . . . . ."

The other morning I heard a four-year-old girl ask her mother, "Why was I born into this world? To go to nursery school?"

Naturally her mother could not honestly say, "Yes, that's right, so off you go." And yet, you could say that people these days *are* born to go to nursery school.

Right up through college people study diligently to learn why they were born. Scholars and philosophers, even if they ruin their lives in the attempt, say they will be satisfied to understand this one thing.

Originally human beings had no purpose. Now, dreaming up some purpose or other, they struggle away trying to find the meaning of life. It is a one-man wrestling match. There is no purpose one has to think about, or go out in search of. You would do well to ask the children whether or not a life without purpose is meaningless.

From the time they enter nursery school, people's sorrows begin. The human being was a happy creature, but he created a hard world and now struggles trying to break out of it.

In nature there is life and death, and nature is joyful.

In human society there is life and death, and people live in sorrow.

# Drifting Clouds and the Illusion of Science

This morning I am washing citrus storage boxes by the river. As I stoop on a flat rock, my hands feel the chill of the autumn river. The red leaves of the sumacs along the river bank stand out against the clear blue autumn sky. I am struck with wonder by the unexpected splendor of the branches against the sky.

Within this casual scene the entire world of experience is present. In the flowing water, the flow of time, the left bank and right bank, the sunshine and shadows, the red leaves and blue sky—all appear within the sacred, silent book of nature. And man is a slender, thinking reed.

Once he inquires what nature is, he then must inquire what that "what" is, and what that human who inquires what that "what" is is. He heads, that is to say, into a world of endless questioning.

In trying to gain a clear understanding of what it is that fills him with wonder, what it is that astonishes him, he has two possible paths. The first is to look deeply into himself, at him who asks the question, "What is nature?"

The second is to examine nature apart from man.

The first path leads to the realm of philosophy and religion. Gazing vacantly, it is not unnatural to see the water as flowing from above to below, but there is no inconsistency in seeing the water as standing still and the bridge as flowing by.

If, on the other hand, following the second path, the scene is divided into a variety of natural phenomena, the water, the speed of the current, the waves, the wind and white clouds, all of these separately become objects of investigation, leading to further questions, which spread out endlessly in all directions. This is the path of science.

The world used to be simple. You merely noticed in passing that you got wet by brushing against the drops of dew while meandering through the meadow. But from the time people undertook to explain this one drop of dew scientifically, they trapped themselves in the endless hell of the intellect.

Water molecules are made up of atoms of hydrogen and oxygen. People once thought that the smallest particles in the world were atoms, but then they found out that there was a nucleus inside the atom. Now they have discovered that within the nucleus there are even tinier particles. Among these nuclear particles there are hundreds of different varieties and no one knows where the examination of this minute world will end.

It is said that the way electrons orbit at ultrahigh speeds within the atom is exactly like the flight of comets within the galaxy. To the atomic physicist the world of elementary particles is a world as vast as the universe itself. Yet it has been shown that in addition to the immediate galaxy in which we live there are countless other galaxies. In the eyes of the cosmologist, then, our entire galaxy becomes infinitesimally small.

The fact is that people who think a drop of water is simple or that a rock is fixed and inert are happy, ignorant fools, and the scientists who know that the drop of water is a great universe and the rock is an active world of elementary particles streaming about like rockets, are clever fools. Looked at simply, this world is real and at hand. Seen as complex, the world becomes frighteningly abstract and distant.

The scientists who rejoiced when rocks were brought back from the moon have less grasp of the moon than the children who sing out, "How old are you, Mr. Moon?" Basho* could apprehend the wonder of nature by watching the reflection of the full moon in the tranquillity of a pond. All the scientists did when they went off into space and stomped around in their spaceboots was to tarnish a bit of the moon's splendor for millions of lovers and children on the earth.

How is it that people think science is beneficial to humanity?

Originally grain was ground into flour in this village by a stone mill which was turned slowly by hand. Then a watermill, which had incomparably greater momentum than the old stone grinder, was built to utilize the power of the river current. Several years ago a dam was constructed to produce hydroelectric power and an electrically powered mill was built.

How do you think this advanced machinery works for the benefit of human beings? In order to grind rice into flour, it is first polished—that is, made into white rice. This means husking the grain, removing the germ and the bran, which are the basis of good health, and keeping the leftovers.** And so the result of this technology is the breaking down of the whole grain into incomplete by-products. If the too easily digestible white rice becomes the daily staple, the

---

*A famous Japanese *haiku* poet (1644-1694).

**In Japanese the character for leftovers—pronounced *kasu*—is composed of radicals meaning "white" and "rice;" the character for bran—*nuka*—is made up of "rice" and "health."

diet lacks nutrients, and dietary supplements become necessary. The water wheel and the milling factory are doing the work of the stomach and intestines, and their consequence is to make these organs lazy.

It is the same with fuel. Crude oil is formed when the tissue of ancient plants buried deep in the earth is transformed by great pressure and heat. This substance is dug out of the desert, sent to a port by pipeline, and then transported by boat to Japan and refined into kerosene and oil at a big refinery.

Which do you think is quicker, warmer, and more convenient, burning this kerosene or branches of cedar or pine from in front of the house?* The fuel is the same plant matter. The oil and kerosene just followed a longer path in getting here.

Now they are saying that the fossil fuels are not enough, and that we need to develop atomic energy. To search out the scarce uranium ore, compress it into radioactive fuel and burn it in a huge nuclear furnace is not as easy as burning dried leaves with a match. Moreover, the hearth fire leaves only ashes, but after a nuclear fire has burned, the radioactive waste remains dangerous for many thousands of years.

The same principle holds in agriculture. Grow a soft, fat rice plant in a flooded field and you get a plant easily attacked by insects and disease. If "improved" seed varieties are used one must rely on the help of chemical insecticides and fertilizer.

On the other hand, if you grow a small, sturdy plant in a healthy environment, these chemicals are unnecessary.

Cultivate a flooded rice field with a plow or tractor and the soil becomes deficient in oxygen, the soil

---

*At the present time much of the world is faced with a shortage of firewood. Implicit in Mr. Fukuoka's argument is the need to plant trees.

More broadly, Mr. Fukuoka is suggesting modest, direct answers to the needs of daily life.

structure is broken down, earthworms and other small animals are destroyed, and the earth becomes hard and lifeless. Once this happens, the field *must* be turned every year.

But if a method is adopted in which the earth cultivates itself naturally, there is no need for a plow or cultivating machine.

After the living soil is burned clean of organic matter and microorganisms, the use of fast-acting fertilizers becomes necessary. If chemical fertilizer is used the rice grows fast and tall, but so do the weeds. Herbicides are then applied and thought to be beneficial.

But if clover is sown with the grain, and all the straw and organic residues are returned to the surface of the field as mulch, crops can be grown without herbicides, chemical fertilizer or prepared compost.

In farming there is little that cannot be eliminated. Prepared fertilizer, herbicide, insecticide, machinery—all are unnecessary. But if a condition is created in which they become necessary, then the power of science is required.

I have demonstrated in my fields that natural farming produces harvests comparable to those of modern scientific agriculture. If the results of a non-active agriculture are comparable to those of science, at a fraction of the investment in labor and resources, then where is the benefit of scientific technology?

## The Theory of Relativity

Looking out into the bright sunlight of the autumn sky, scanning the surrounding fields, I was amazed. In every field but mine there was a rice harvesting machine or combine running around. In the last three years, this village has changed beyond recognition.

As one might expect, the youths on the mountain do not envy the changeover to mechanization. They enjoy the quiet, peaceful harvest with the old hand sickle.

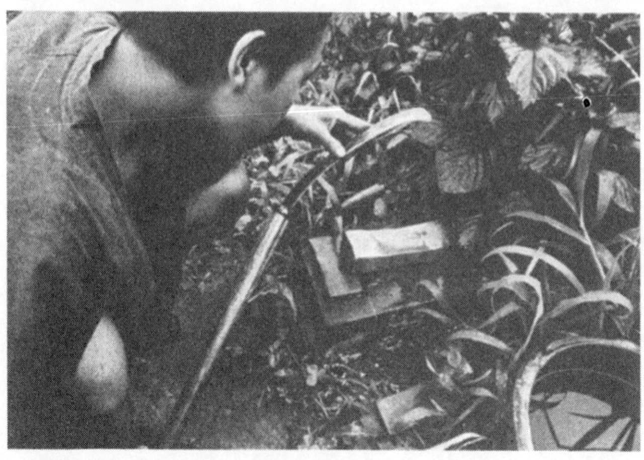

Sharpening a long-handled scythe.

That night as we were finishing the evening meal, I recalled over tea how, long ago in this village, in the days when the farmers were turning the fields by hand, one man began to use a cow. He was very proud of the ease and speed with which he could finish the laborious job of plowing. Twenty years ago when the first mechanical cultivator made its appearance, the villagers all got together and debated seriously which was better, the cow or the machine. In two or three years it became clear that plowing by machine was faster, and without looking beyond considerations of time and convenience, the farmers abandoned their draft animals. The inducement was simply to finish the job more quickly than the farmer in the next field.

The farmer does not realize that he has merely become a factor in modern agriculture's equation of increasing speed and efficiency. He lets the farm equipment salesman do all the figuring for him.

Originally people would look into a starry night sky and feel awe at the vastness of the universe. Now questions of time and space are left entirely to the consideration of scientists.

It is said that Einstein was given the Nobel Prize in physics in deference to the incomprehensibility of his theory of relativity. If his theory had explained clearly the phenomenon of relativity in the world and thus released humanity from the confines of time and space, bringing about a more pleasant and peaceful world, it would have been commendable. His explanation is bewildering, however, and it caused people to think that the world is complex beyond all possible understanding. A citation for "disturbing the peace of the human spirit" should have been awarded instead.

In nature, the world of relativity does not exist. The idea of relative phenomena is a structure given to experience by the human intellect. Other animals live in a world of undivided reality. To the extent that one lives in the relative world of the intellect, one loses sight of time that is beyond time and of space that is beyond space.

"You might be wondering why I have this habit of picking on the scientists all the time," I said, pausing to take a sip of tea. The youths looked up smiling, faces glowing and flickering in the firelight. "It's because the role of the scientist in society is analogous to the role of discrimination in your own minds."

# A Village Without War and Peace

A snake seizes a frog in its mouth and slips away into the grass. A girl screams. A brave lad bares his feelings of loathing and flings a rock at the snake. The others laugh. I turn to the boy who threw the stone: "What do you think that's going to accomplish?"

The hawk hunts the snake. The wolf attacks the hawk. A human kills the wolf, and later succumbs to a tuberculosis virus. Bacteria breed in the remains of the human, and other animals, grasses, and trees thrive on the nutrients made available by the bacteria's activity. Insects attack the trees, the frog eats the insects.

Animals, plants, microorganisms—all are part of the cycle of life. Maintaining a suitable balance, they live a naturally regulated existence. People may choose to view this world either as a model of strong consuming weak, or of co-existence and mutual benefit. Either way, it is an arbitrary interpretation which causes wind and waves, brings about disorder and confusion.

Adults think the frog is deserving of pity, and feeling compassion for its death, despise the snake. This feeling may seem to be natural, just a matter of course, but is this what it really is?

One youth said, "If life is seen as a contest in which the strong consume the weak, the face of the earth becomes a hell of carnage and destruction. But it is unavoidable that the weak should be sacrificed so that the strong may live. That the strong win and survive and the weak die out is a rule of nature. After the passage of millions of years, the creatures now living on the earth have been victorious in the struggle for life. You could say that the survival of the fittest is a providence of nature."

Said a second youth, "That's how it appears to the winners, anyway. The way I see it, this world is one of co-existence and mutual benefit. At the foot of the grain in this field, clover, and so many varieties of grasses and weeds are living mutually beneficial lives. Ivy winds around the trees; moss and lichen live attached to the tree's trunk and branches. Ferns spread beneath the forest canopy. Birds and frogs, plants, insects, small animals, bacteria, fungi—all creatures perform essential roles and benefit from one another's existence."

A third spoke, "The earth is a world of the strong consuming the weak, and also one of co-existence. The stronger creatures take no more food than necessary; though they attack other creatures, the overall balance of nature is maintained. The providence of nature is an ironclad rule, preserving peace and order upon the earth."

Three people and three points of view. I met all three opinions with a flat denial.

The world itself never asks whether it is based upon a principle of competition or of cooperation. When seen from the relative perspective of the human intellect, there are those who are strong and there are those who are weak, there is large and there is small.

Now there is no one who doubts that this relative outlook exists, but if we were to suppose that the relativity of human perception is mistaken—for

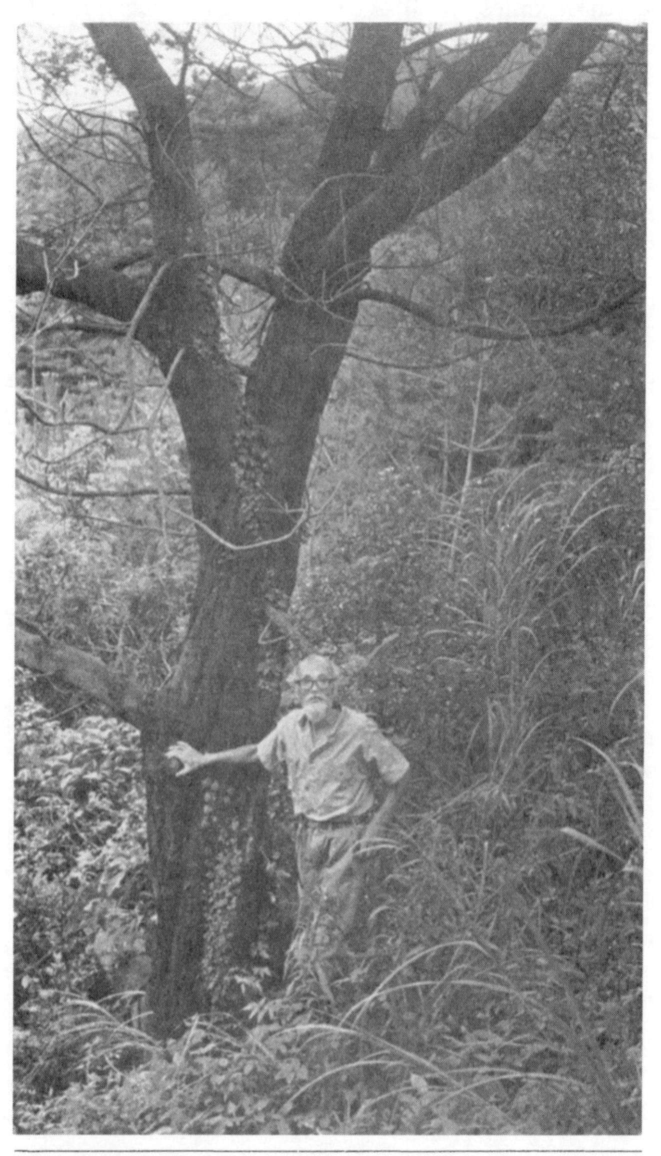

"In nature, the world of relativity does not exist."

example, that there is no big and no small, no up or down—if we say there is no such standpoint at all, human values and judgment would collapse.

"Isn't that way of seeing the world an empty flight of the imagination? In reality, there are large countries and small countries. If there is poverty and plenty, strong and weak, inevitably there will be disputes, and consequently, winners and losers. Couldn't you say, rather, that these relative perceptions and the resulting emotions are human and therefore natural, that they are a unique privilege of being human?"

Other animals fight but do not make war. If you say that making war, which depends upon ideas of strong and weak, is humanity's special "privilege," then life is a farce. Not knowing this farce to be a farce—there lies the human tragedy.

The ones who live peacefully in a world of no contradictions and no distinctions are infants. They perceive light and dark, strong and weak, but make no judgments. Even though the snake and the frog exist, the child has no understanding of strong and weak. The original joy of life is there, but the fear of death is yet to appear.

The love and hate which arise in the adult's eyes originally were not two separate things. They are the same thing as seen from the front and from the back. Love gives substance to hate. If you turn the coin of love over, it becomes hate. Only by penetrating to an absolute world of no aspects, is it possible to avoid becoming lost in the duality of the phenomenal world.

People distinguish between Self and Other. To the extent that the ego exists, to the extent that there is an "other," people will not be relieved from love and hatred. The heart that loves the wicked ego creates the hated enemy. For humans, the first and greatest enemy is the Self that they hold so dear.

People choose to attack or to defend. In the ensuing struggle they accuse one another of instigating conflict. It is like clapping your hands and then arguing about which is making the sound, the right hand or the left. In all contentions there is neither right nor wrong, neither good nor bad. All conscious distinctions arise at the same time and all are mistaken.

To build a fortress is wrong from the start. Even though he gives the excuse that it is for the city's defense, the castle is the outcome of the ruling lord's personality, and exerts a coercive force on the surrounding area. Saying he is afraid of attack and that fortification is for the town's protection, the bully stocks up weapons and puts the key in the door.

The act of defense is already an attack. Weapons for self-defense always give a pretext to those who instigate wars. The calamity of war comes from the strengthening and magnifying of empty distinctions of self/other, strong/weak, attack/defense.

There is no other road to peace than for all people to depart from the castle gate of relative perception, go down into the meadow, and return to the heart of non-active nature. That is, sharpening the sickle instead of the sword.

The farmers of long ago were a peaceful people, but now they are arguing with Australia about meat, quarreling with Russia over fish, and dependent on America for wheat and soybeans.

I feel as if we in Japan are living in the shadow of a big tree, and there is no place more dangerous to be during a thunderstorm than under a big tree. And there could be nothing more foolish than taking shelter under a "nuclear umbrella" which will be the first target in the next war. Now we are tilling the earth beneath that dark umbrella. I feel as though a crisis is approaching from both inside and out.

Get rid of the aspects of inside and outside. Farmers everywhere in the world are at root the same farmers. Let us say that the key to peace lies close to the earth.

# The One-Straw Revolution

Among the young people who come to these mountain huts, there are those, poor in body and spirit, who have given up all hope. I am only an old farmer who grieves that he cannot even provide them with a pair of sandals—but there is still one thing I *can* give them.

One straw.

I picked up some straw from in front of the hut and said, "From just this one straw a revolution could begin."

"With the destruction of mankind at hand, you can still hope to cling to a straw?" one youth asked, with a touch of bitterness in his voice.

This straw appears small and light, and most people do not know how really weighty it is. If people knew the true value of this straw a human revolution could occur which would become powerful enough to move the country and the world.

When I was a child there was a man who lived near Inuyose Pass. All he seemed to do was to pack charcoal on horseback two miles or so along the road from the top of the mountain to the port of Gunchu. And yet he became rich. If you ask how, people will tell you that on his trip homeward from the port he gathered the discarded straw horseshoes and the manure by the side of the road and put them onto his field. His motto was: "Treat one strand of straw as important and never take a useless step." It made him a wealthy man.

"Even if you burned the straw, I don't think it could kindle a spark to start a revolution."

A gentle breeze rustled through the orchard trees, sunlight flickering among the green leaves. I began to talk about using straw in growing rice.

It has been nearly forty years since I realized how important straw could be in growing rice and barley. At that time, passing an old rice field in Kochi Prefecture which had been left unused and uncultivated for many years, I saw healthy young rice sprouting up through a tangle of weeds and straw which had accumulated on the field's surface. After working on the implications of that for many years, I came out advocating a completely new method of rice and barley growing.

Believing that this was a natural and revolutionary way of farming, I wrote about it in books and magazines, and spoke of it on television and radio dozens of times.

It seems a very simple thing, but farmers are so set in their thinking about how straw should be used, that it is unlikely that they will accept change easily. Spreading fresh straw on a field can be risky because rice blast and stem rot are diseases always present in rice straw. In the past, these diseases have caused great damage, and this is one of the main reasons that farmers have always turned the straw into compost before putting it back onto the field. Long ago, careful disposal of rice straw was commonly practiced as a countermeasure against blast disease, and there were times in Hokkaido when the wholesale burning of straw was required by law.

Stem borers also enter the straw to pass the winter. To prevent an infestation of these insects, farmers used to compost the straw carefully all winter long to be sure that it would be completely decomposed by the following spring. That is why Japanese farmers have always kept their fields so neat and tidy. The practical knowledge of everyday life was that if farmers left straw lying around, they would be punished by heaven for their negligence.

After years of experimentation, even technical experts have now confirmed my theory that spreading fresh straw on the field six months before seeding is completely safe. This overturned all previous ideas on the subject. But it is going to be a long while before the farmers become receptive to using straw in this manner.

Farmers have been working for centuries to try to increase the production of compost. The Ministry of Agriculture used to give incentive pay to encourage compost production, and competitive compost exhibitions were held as annual events. Farmers came to believe in compost as though it were the protective deity of the soil. Now again there is a movement to make more compost, "better" compost, with earthworms and "compost-starter." There is no reason to expect an easy acceptance of my suggestion that prepared compost is unnecessary, that all you have to do is scatter fresh unshredded straw across the field.

In traveling up to Tokyo, looking out the window of the Tokaido train, I have seen the transformation of the Japanese countryside. Looking at the winter fields, the appearance of which has completely changed in ten years, I feel an anger I cannot express. The former landscape of neat fields of green barley, Chinese milk vetch, and blooming rape plants is nowhere to be seen. Instead, half-burned straw is piled roughly in heaps and left soaking in the rain. That this straw is being neglected is proof of the disorder of modern farming. The barrenness of these fields reveals the barrenness of the farmer's spirit. It challenges the responsibility of government leaders, and clearly points out the absence of a wise agricultural policy.

The man who several years ago talked about a "merciful end" to the growing of winter grain, of its "death by the side of the road"—what does he think now when he sees these empty fields? Seeing the barren fields of wintertime Japan, I can remain patient no longer. With this straw, I, by myself, will begin a revolution!

The youths who had been listening silently were now roaring with laughter.

"A one-man revolution! Tomorrow let's get a big sack of barley, rice, and clover seed and take off, carrying it on our shoulders, like Okuninushi-no-mikoto,* and broadcast seeds all over the fields of Tokaido."

"That's not a one-man revolution," I laughed, "it's a *one-straw* revolution!"

Stepping out of the hut into the afternoon sunlight, I paused for a moment and gazed at the surrounding orchard trees laden with ripening fruit, and at the chickens scratching in the weeds and clover. I then began my familiar descent to the fields.

---

*The legendary Japanese god of healing who travels around tossing good fortune from a large sack which he carries over his shoulder.

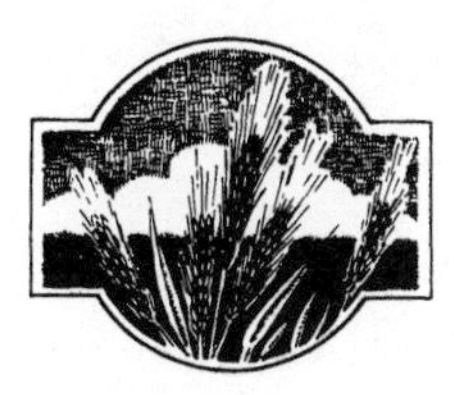

To my readers,

There is nowhere better than this world. Years ago I realized that we human beings are good just as we are and I set out to enjoy my life. I took a carefree road back to nature, free from human knowledge and effort. Since then fifty years of my life have flown away. I have had some successes, but also failures. Many of my youthful dreams remain unfulfilled. I know my time here on earth is limited.

I am retired now and live in a mountain hut in the orchard. I have closed my farm to the public so that I can better cherish the time left to me. The best part of living a retired life on the mountain, isolated from news of the outside world, is that I have a different sense of time. I hope, as the days go by, that I will be able to experience a day as a year. Then, like the tribal people I met in Somalia, I will not know how old I am.

These days I try to imagine that I am one hundred years old...or even two hundred. I hope that when I pass away my mind and body will still be in good condition. When I go to the fields or the orchard I say to myself: make no promises, forget about yesterday, do not think about tomorrow, put sincere effort into each day's work and leave no footprints here on earth. I am happy simply to work joyfully on my farm, which to me is the Garden of Eden. The way of natural farming is forever uncompleted. Nature can never be understood or improved upon by human effort. In the end, to become one with nature, to live with God, one cannot help others or even receive help from them. We can only walk our paths alone.

Great road without a gate, I see no one
Peace in Heaven but a murmur on the land
Who makes the wandering wind?
To the left, to the right
Attack and defend
Not knowing good from bad
A fan blows to both sides, making the same
  shambles

As I walk alone in the garden I see a temporary hut
A day is a hundred years
Daikon and mustard are in full bloom
Dimly the moon shines in the year two thousand
Having tried my best in this world, I now begin my
  journey to another world
A transient voyage to who knows where

*Early spring, 1986*

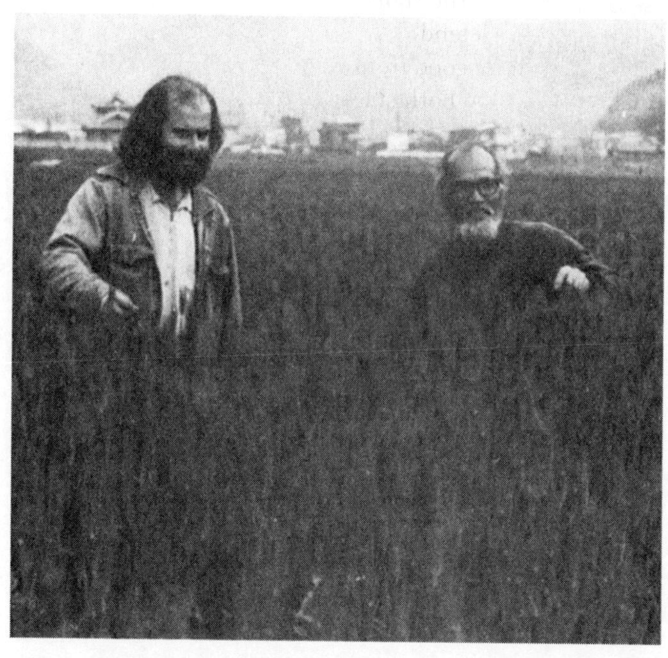

*The One-Straw Revolution was designed and produced by Jack Shoemaker and George Mattingly, and typeset in Trump Mediaeval by Bob Sibley, in Berkeley, 1977-78.*

## OTHER NEW YORK REVIEW CLASSICS

*For a complete list of titles, visit www.nyrb.com or write to:*
*Catalog Requests, NYRB, 435 Hudson Street, New York, NY 10014*

**HENRY ADAMS** The Jeffersonian Transformation
**RENATA ADLER** Speedboat*
**ROBERT AICKMAN** Compulsory Games*
**CÉLESTE ALBARET** Monsieur Proust
**KINGSLEY AMIS** Lucky Jim*
**U.R. ANANTHAMURTHY** Samskara: A Rite for a Dead Man*
**IVO ANDRIĆ** Omer Pasha Latas*
**W.H. AUDEN (EDITOR)** The Living Thoughts of Kierkegaard
**ERICH AUERBACH** Dante: Poet of the Secular World
**EVE BABITZ** I Used to Be Charming: The Rest of Eve Babitz*
**J.A. BAKER** The Peregrine
**S. JOSEPHINE BAKER** Fighting for Life*
**HONORÉ DE BALZAC** The Human Comedy: Selected Stories*
**SYBILLE BEDFORD** A Visit to Don Otavio: A Mexican Journey*
**FRANS G. BENGTSSON** The Long Ships*
**WALTER BENJAMIN** The Storyteller Essays*
**ALEXANDER BERKMAN** Prison Memoirs of an Anarchist
**MIRON BIAŁOSZEWSKI** A Memoir of the Warsaw Uprising*
**ADOLFO BIOY CASARES** The Invention of Morel
**LESLEY BLANCH** Journey into the Mind's Eye: Fragments of an Autobiography*
**RONALD BLYTHE** Akenfield: Portrait of an English Village*
**EMMANUEL BOVE** My Friends*
**SIR THOMAS BROWNE** Religio Medici and Urne-Buriall*
**DAVID R. BUNCH** Moderan*
**ROBERT BURTON** The Anatomy of Melancholy
**MATEI CALINESCU** The Life and Opinions of Zacharias Lichter*
**CAMARA LAYE** The Radiance of the King
**J.L. CARR** A Month in the Country*
**LEONORA CARRINGTON** Down Below*
**EILEEN CHANG** Little Reunions*
**JOAN CHASE** During the Reign of the Queen of Persia*
**ELLIOTT CHAZE** Black Wings Has My Angel*
**UPAMANYU CHATTERJEE** English, August: An Indian Story
**FRANÇOIS-RENÉ DE CHATEAUBRIAND** Memoirs from Beyond the Grave, 1768–1800
**NIRAD C. CHAUDHURI** The Autobiography of an Unknown Indian
**ANTON CHEKHOV** Peasants and Other Stories
**JEAN-PAUL CLÉBERT** Paris Vagabond*
**D.G. COMPTON** The Continuous Katherine Mortenhoe
**BARBARA COMYNS** The Juniper Tree*
**ALBERT COSSERY** The Jokers*
**ASTOLPHE DE CUSTINE** Letters from Russia*
**JÓZEF CZAPSKI** Inhuman Land: Searching for the Truth in Soviet Russia, 1941-1942 *
**ELIZABETH DAVID** A Book of Mediterranean Food
**L.J. DAVIS** A Meaningful Life*
**MARIA DERMOÛT** The Ten Thousand Things
**TIBOR DÉRY** Niki: The Story of a Dog
**ANTONIO DI BENEDETTO** Zama*

* *Also available as an electronic book.*

**ALFRED DÖBLIN** Berlin Alexanderplatz*
**JEAN D'ORMESSON** The Glory of the Empire: A Novel, A History*
**CHARLES DUFF** A Handbook on Hanging
**BRUCE DUFFY** The World As I Found It*
**DAPHNE DU MAURIER** Don't Look Now: Stories
**ELAINE DUNDY** The Dud Avocado*
**G.B. EDWARDS** The Book of Ebenezer Le Page*
**JOHN EHLE** The Land Breakers*
**EURIPIDES** Grief Lessons: Four Plays; translated by Anne Carson
**J.G. FARRELL** Troubles*
**ELIZA FAY** Original Letters from India
**FÉLIX FÉNÉON** Novels in Three Lines*
**M.I. FINLEY** The World of Odysseus
**BENJAMIN FONDANE** Existential Monday: Philosophical Essays*
**SANFORD FRIEDMAN** Conversations with Beethoven*
**MAVIS GALLANT** Paris Stories*
**GABRIEL GARCÍA MÁRQUEZ** Clandestine in Chile: The Adventures of Miguel Littín
**LEONARD GARDNER** Fat City*
**WILLIAM H. GASS** In the Heart of the Heart of the Country and Other Stories*
**NATALIA GINZBURG** Family Lexicon*
**FRANÇOISE GILOT** Life with Picasso*
**JEAN GIONO** Hill*
**JEAN GIONO** A King Alone*
**P.V. GLOB** The Bog People: Iron-Age Man Preserved
**ALICE GOODMAN** History Is Our Mother: Three Libretti*
**PAUL GOODMAN** Growing Up Absurd: Problems of Youth in the Organized Society*
**A.C. GRAHAM** Poems of the Late T'ang
**HENRY GREEN** Nothing*
**HENRY GREEN** Party Going*
**VASILY GROSSMAN** Life and Fate*
**VASILY GROSSMAN** Stalingrad*
**PETER HANDKE** Short Letter, Long Farewell
**THORKILD HANSEN** Arabia Felix: The Danish Expedition of 1761–1767*
**ELIZABETH HARDWICK** The Collected Essays of Elizabeth Hardwick*
**L.P. HARTLEY** The Go-Between*
**NATHANIEL HAWTHORNE** Twenty Days with Julian & Little Bunny by Papa
**ALFRED HAYES** My Face for the World to See*
**PAUL HAZARD** The Crisis of the European Mind: 1680–1715*
**ALICE HERDAN-ZUCKMAYER** The Farm in the Green Mountains*
**WOLFGANG HERRNDORF** Sand*
**GILBERT HIGHET** Poets in a Landscape
**RUSSELL HOBAN** Turtle Diary*
**YOEL HOFFMANN** The Sound of the One Hand: 281 Zen Koans with Answers*
**RICHARD HOLMES** Shelley: The Pursuit*
**GEOFFREY HOUSEHOLD** Rogue Male*
**BOHUMIL HRABAL** Dancing Lessons for the Advanced in Age*
**DOROTHY B. HUGHES** In a Lonely Place*
**RICHARD HUGHES** A High Wind in Jamaica*
**INTIZAR HUSAIN** Basti*
**YASUSHI INOUE** Tun-huang*
**HENRY JAMES** The New York Stories of Henry James*
**TOVE JANSSON** Fair Play *
**TOVE JANSSON** The Summer Book*